Laboratory Manual to accompany Pharmacy Technician

Practice and Procedures

Gail Orum-Alexander, PharmD.

*Charles Drew University of Medicine and Science
Dean, College of Science and Health*

James J. Mizner, Jr., BS Pharmacy, MBA, RPh.

*ACT College
Pharmacy Technician and AHT Program Director
Arlington, VA*

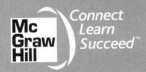

*Connect
Learn
Succeed*™

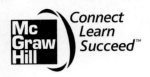

LABORATORY MANUAL TO ACCOMPANY PHARMACY TECHNICIAN:
PRACTICE AND PROCEDURES, FIRST EDITION
Gail G. Orum-Alexander and James Mizner

Published by McGraw-Hill, a business unit of The McGraw-Hill Companies, Inc., 1221 Avenue of the Americas, New York, NY 10020. Copyright © 2011 by The McGraw-Hill Companies, Inc. All rights reserved.

1 2 3 4 5 6 7 8 9 0 WDQ/WDQ 0

ISBN   978-0-07-320269-3
MHID   0-07-320269-X

Credits: The credits section for this book begins on page 209 and is considered an extension of the copyright page.

WARNING NOTICE: The clinical procedures, medicines, dosages, and other matters described in this publication are based upon research of current literature and consultation with knowledgeable persons in the field. The procedures and matters described in this text reflect currently accepted clinical practice. However, this information cannot and should not be relied upon as necessarily applicable to a given individual's case. Accordingly, each person must be separately diagnosed to discern the patient's unique circumstances. Likewise, the manufacturer's package insert for current drug product information should be consulted before administering any drug. Publisher disclaims all liability for any inaccuracies, omissions, misuse, or misunderstanding of the information contained in this publication. Publisher cautions that this publication is not intended as a substitute for the professional judgment of trained medical personnel.

www.mhhe.com

Contents

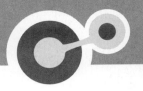

Preface

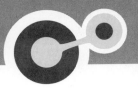

When you visit your local pharmacy to refill a prescription, whom do you meet first? In most situations, you will meet a very valuable member of the pharmacy team, the pharmacy technician.

According to the U.S. Department of Labor Statistics Occupational Outlook, 2008–2009, employment for pharmacy technicians is expected to increase much faster than the average through 2016, and job opportunities are expected to be good.

Due to this rapid growth and increased need for pharmacy technicians, the *Pharmacy Technician: Practice and Procedures* text has evolved. This rapid growth and increased need for pharmacy technicians is based upon two primary factors:

- Increased use of medications
- Shortage of registered pharmacists

The aging population and the advancement and augmented use of prescription medications have consequently increased the need for dispensing of medications whether it is in long-term care, acute care, or outpatient pharmacy practice. Although automation and centralization of services was predicted to decrease the need for registered pharmacists the amplified use of medications by the population has outweighed these factors.

Pharmacists are in high demand and the shortage of pharmacists is expected to increase over the next decade. Pharmacists require well-trained pharmacy technicians to assist them with basic tasks, so they can be available to perform counseling and other higher-level functions. In order for pharmacy technicians to be well trained, they need exceptional educational materials—thus the magnified need for McGraw-Hill's *Laboratory Manual to accompany Pharmacy Technician: Practice and Procedures.*

Student-Based Learning

With McGraw-Hill's *Laboratory Manual to Accompany Pharmacy Technician: Practice and Procedures* text, pharmacy technician training is brought to a new level. The easy-to-understand language and format was created to make this challenging content interesting as well as comprehensive. Students in the pharmacy technician program need to be stimulated and motivated to learn the necessary information to enter the field.

Organization

The laboratory manual is intended for entry-level as well as seasoned learners who want to prepare themselves for the pharmacy technician profession. In addition to **learning outcomes** and a **correlation to the knowledge statements for the Pharmacy Technician Certification Board** exam, each chapter includes many other essential features.

The *Laboratory Manual to accompany Pharmacy Technician: Practice and Procedures* provides students with the opportunity to test their recall of text concepts and applications. The *Laboratory Manual* features include:

- **Learning Outcomes**
- **Test Your Knowledge**
  - Multiple choice questions
  - True/false questions
  - Matching
- **Apply Your Knowledge**
  - Research information on the Web
  - Answer questions that require critical thinking
- **Practice Your Knowledge**
  - Complete a research task
  - Complete a laboratory procedure
- **Calculation Corner**
  - Work out solutions to common pharmacy calculation problems
- **Pharmacy Facts—Research**
  - Use reference material to research concepts and topics in pharmacy.
- **Did You Know?**
  - Read about a bit of pharmacy trivia and interesting data.

Teaching and Learning Supplements

You will find many useful teaching and learning supplements with McGraw-Hill's *Pharmacy Technician: Practice and Procedures* and its accompanying *Laboratory Manual.* These supplements create a complete package for to-day's learner whether they are learning on the job, on their own, through distance education, or in the typical classroom setting.

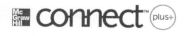

- **McGraw-Hill *Connect Plus*** is a Web-based assignment and assessment platform that gives students the means to better connect with their coursework, with their instructors, and with the important concepts that they will need to know for success now and in the future. With *Connect Plus* instructors can deliver assignments, quizzes, and tests easily online. Students can practice important skills at their own pace and on their own schedule. With *Connect Plus*, students also get 24/7 online access to an eBook—an online edition of the text—to aid them in successfully completing their work, wherever and whenever they choose.

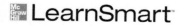

- **McGraw-Hill LearnSmart: Pharmacology** is a diagnostic learning system that determines the level of student knowledge, then feeds the student appropriate content. Students learn faster and study more efficiently.

As a student works within the system, LearnSmart develops a personal learning path adapted to what the student has learned and retained. LearnSmart is also able to recommend additional study resources to help the student master topics.

In addition to being an innovative, outstanding study tool, Learn-Smart has features for instructors. There is a Course Gauge where the instructor can see exactly what students have accomplished as well as a built-in assessment tool for graded assignments.

Students and instructors will be able to access LearnSmart anywhere via a web browser. And for students on the go, it will also be available through any iPhone or iPod Touch.

- **Student Applications CD-ROM** accompanies the main text. This CD assists the student in learning the content presented in the textbook as well as preparing for their certification test. This easy to use CD promotes critical thinking, learning of skills and provides drill and practice activities all in one.

  Over 75 *Topic Specific Activities* are correlated to the textbook learning objectives as well as the ASHP Modules and PTCB Knowledge Statements. These activities include videos, photos, matching, drag and drop, and completion exercises. Each activity is graded and student scores are tracked on any writable media. Results can be emailed to the instructor and/or printed to be included in the student's portfolio. *Interactive Games* require knowledge of the chapter content, a good memory and an interest in having fun while learning. Games can be used for enrichment, reinforcement, and/or review and support the current edutainment trend of today's high tech learner.

- **Spin the Wheel Game** A learning game that infuses a bit of chance; this game can be used for classroom or student review. Users can select one or multiple chapters. Play the game with one, two, three, or four players or teams. Questions are created from the chapter objectives. This game can be used for classroom or individual review. It will allow the user to choose the chapter and/or chapters they would like to review and split the students into teams for classroom or small group activity. (The Instructor Productivity CD allows the instructor to change, add or delete questions for this game.)

- **Brand Generic Concentration Game** An interactive matching game that helps the student learn common Brand and Generic drug names as well as drug categories. The user matches drugs to uncover a picture. With each match, part of the picture is revealed and you must answer a question related to the picture for extra points. The computer monitors the number of matches. All matches must be completed before the picture is revealed and the student can play again. Each time the puzzle is created the medications are randomized from a master list so no two games are alike. The game is designed for two players or teams.

- **Pharm Tech Challenge** A jeopardy-like game that provides lots of fun for up to three players. An *audio glossary, brand-generic flash cards, presentation reviews, key terms quizzes,* and *chapter tests* round out the educational content and provide additional multiple review and learning activities for the user.

- **Instructor Resource CD-ROM** includes easy-to-use resources for class preparation. The CD includes the following:
    - PowerPoint® presentations with *Apply Your Knowledge* questions and Instructor notes.
    - McGraw-Hill's EZTest Test Generator with over 500 questions and answer rationales and correlations to PTCB and ASHP competencies. The flexible electronic testing program allows instructors to create tests from book-specific items. It accommodates a wide range of question types, and instructors may add their own questions. Multiple versions of the test can be created and any test can be exported for use with course management systems such as WebCT, BlackBoard, or PageOut. EZTest Online gives instructors a chance to easily administer.
    - EZTest-created exams and quizzes online. EZTest Online is available for Windows and Macintosh environments.
    - Electronic resources including answers to the textbook questions, lesson plans, and correlation charts to PTCB and ASHP.
    - Image Bank with selected figures from the textbook that can be utilized in classroom presentations, handouts, or questions.

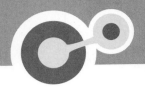

Gail Orum-Alexander

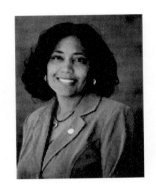

Gail Orum-Alexander has a Doctor of Pharmacy degree from the University of Southern California, School of Pharmacy and is a registered pharmacist in the state of California. She is the Dean of the College of Science and Health at Charles R. Drew University of Medicine and Science. She also serves as director of the Pharmacy Technology Program. She has published and reviewed articles on the pharmacologic management of obesity and obesity in children and adolescents.

Dr. Orum-Alexander is actively involved in local and national organizations, as well as community programs that focus on minority health issues. She is a member of the American Society of Health-System Pharmacists and has served as a site visitor for pharmacy technician program accreditation. She is a member of the Pharmacy Technician Educators Council and has served as an item writer for the Pharmacy Technician Certification Examination. Her honors include Most Outstanding Faculty Award, Charles R. Drew University, College of Science and Health (1997 and 1998), Recognition Awards from Physician Assistant Students (2002 and 2003), and the Outstanding Faculty Service Award, Charles R. Drew University, (2004).

Dr. Orum-Alexander resides in Alhambra, California, and enjoys reading, needle arts, and walking.

James Mizner

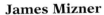

Jim Mizner received a BS in Pharmacy from Duquesne University and an MBA from Keller Graduate School of Business. He is a licensed pharmacist in the state of Virginia with experience in both retail and hospital pharmacy. He is the director for the Pharmacy Technician and the Allied Health Technology Programs at ACT College located in Rosslyn, Virginia. He is also an on-line adjunct pharmacy technician professor for National University.

In addition to teaching, Mizner is a pharmacy technician program specialist for both the Accrediting Bureau of Health Education Schools (ABHES) and the Ohio Board of Regents. In his spare time, he studies Tae Kwon Do with his son. He resides in Reston, Virginia, with his wife and son.

Acknowledgments

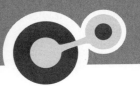

For insightful reviews, helpful suggestions, and information, we would like to acknowledge the following:

Robert W. Aanonsen, CPhT
Platt College

Lori Andrews
Ivy Tech Community College

Trisha Autry, CPhT
Clover Park Technical College

Sybil Barnes
Long Technical College

Nora Chan, Pharm D
City College of San Francisco

Chris P. Crigger, CPhT
San Antonio College

Charleen A. Daniel
*Sixth Avenue Medical Pharmacy
    Pharmacy Technician/Trainer
    Washington State Pharmacy
    Association Technician
    Representative*

Karen Davis, CPhT
Consultant

Cathy L. Dease, BS, MS, MBA
*Pharmacy Branch
Army Medical Department Center
    and School*

Lynn Egler, RMA, AHI, CPhT
Medical Coordinator/Externship
    Coordinator
Dorsey Schools

Donna Fresnilla, BA
*Community College of Rhode
    Island*

Jill M. Frost, BS, CPhT
Tennessee Technology Center

Coelle Lynette Harper Deaton, BSE
Career Centers of Texas–Fort Worth

Linda Hart, CPhT, AS/Pt
High-Tech Institute

Gary W. Haworth, MEd, RPh
Linn-Benton Community College

Michael M. Hayter, Pharm. D., MBA
*Virginia Highlands Community
    College*

A. G. Hirst, AA, BA
North Georgia Technical College

Eddy van Hunnik, PhD
Gibbs College of Boston

Linda C. Kelley, CPhT
MedVance Institute

Mindy Koppel, CPhT
CHI Institute Southampton

Barbara Lacher, BS
*North Dakota State College of
    Science*

Danny D. Lame, MA, BA, AA
Platt College

James P. Lear, AA
National Institute of Technology

Tonya Lewis, CPhT
Georgia Medical Institute

Barbara A. Lipp, CPhT
Bryman College

Jemey Martin
Georgia Medical Institute

Michelle C. McCranie, CPhT
Ogeechee Technical College

Janet McGregor Liles, BS
Arkansas State University–Beebe

Earl R. McKinstry, RPh, MS
Western Dakota Technical Institute

Tara G. McManaway, MDiv, LPC
ALPS (WV), LMT (WV) CMT
(MD)
College of Southern Maryland

Michael Meir, MD
Director HIT
TCI College

Salvatore J. Monopoli, DPM
The Cittone Institute

Nancy L. Needham, MEd, CPhT
American Career College

Hieu T. Nguyen, BS
Western Career College

Joshua Owens, BA
*Bridgerland Applied Technology
College*

Christina Rauberts Conklin, AA,
RMA
Florida Metropolitan University

David R. Reiter, AS
Pueblo Community College

Phil Rushing, BSPharm
Community Care College

Patricia A. Schommer, MA, CPhT
National American University

Douglas Scribner, BA, CPhT
TVI Community College

Susan M. Shorey, BA, MA
Valley Career College

Karen A. Smith, CPhT
Bryman College

Jason P. Sparks, BA, CPhT
Austin Community College

Cynthia J. Steffen, RPh
Milwaukee Area Technical College

Cardiece Sylvan, CPhT.
*Pharmacy Technician Program
Director*
MedVance Institute

Lisa R. Thompson, CPhT
MedVance Institute

Joseph A. Tinervia, CPhT, MBA
*Tulsa Job Corps Pharmacy
Technician*

Sandi Tschritter, BA, CPhT
Spokane Community College

Cindy Turner, CPhT
Western Career College

Pedro A. Valentin, CPhT, BBA
Columbus Technical College

Ray Vellenga, RPh, MS
Century College

Janice Vermiglio-Smith, RN, MS,
PhD
Central Arizona College

Marvin L. Walker, Jr., AAS
Austin Community College

Judy S. Weisbard, MPA, CPhT
Chaffey College

Denise A. Wilfong, MHS, NREMT-P
Western Carolina University

Marsha L. Wilson, MA, BS, MEd
Clarian Health

Richard L. Witt, BS
Allegany College of Maryland

Dr. Betty Yarhi, Pharm D, BS
ACT College

Hwa H. Yeon, AA
Everest College

The Pharmacy Technician

Unit 1

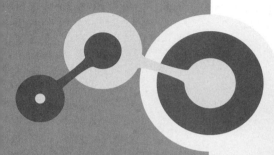

1

Overview, Practice Settings, and Organizations

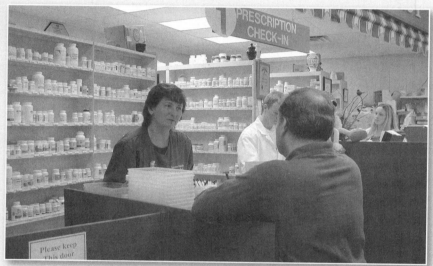

Learning Outcomes

Upon completion of this laboratory chapter, you will be able to:

L-1-1 Explain and demonstrate characteristics associated with a pharmacy technician.

L-1-2 Explain the role of the pharmacy technician as it exists today in the practice of pharmacy.

L-1-3 Differentiate between the duties of a pharmacy technician and a pharmacist.

L-1-4 Demonstrate an appreciation of the evolvement of the practice of pharmacy from the beginning of humanity to its present-day form.

L-1-5 Differentiate between certification, licensure, and registration with a state board of pharmacy.

L-1-6 Describe the various types of training pharmacy technicians may experience in the preparation of their career.

(Continued)

PTCB

In preparation for the certification examination, you should understand and perform activities associated with the following PTCB Knowledge Statements:

Domain I. Assisting the Pharmacist in Serving Patients

Knowledge of pharmaceutical, medical, and legal developments that impact on the practice of pharmacy (2)

Domain III. Participation in the Administration and Management of Pharmacy Practice

Knowledge of required operational licenses and certificates (6)

Knowledge of roles and responsibilities of pharmacists, pharmacy technicians, and other pharmacy employees (7)

Knowledge of professional standards for personnel, facilities equipment, and supplies (9)

Introduction to Pharmacy(L-1-3)

Pharmacy is the art and science of preparing and dispensing medications and providing drug-related information to the public. It involves interpreting of prescriptions and medication orders; compounding, labeling, and dispensing of drugs and devices; drug product selection and drug utilization review; patient monitoring and intervention; and provision of cognitive services related to the use of medications and devices. According to the American Pharmacists Association, or APhA (formerly the American Pharmaceutical Association), the mission of pharmacy is to serve society as "the profession responsible for the appropriate use of medications, devices and services to achieve optimal therapeutic outcomes."

Learning Outcomes *(Cont'd)*

L-1-7 Differentiate between the various pharmacy settings where a pharmacy technician may practice and the responsibilities found in each setting.

Test Your Knowledge

Multiple Choice Questions

Answer the following multiple choice questions. When you have finished, check your answers and then review those areas that need improvement.

1. Which of the following is *not* a role of the pharmacist?(L-1-3)
   a. Collecting information from patients regarding their health
   b. Counseling patients regarding use of their medication
   c. Providing information to health care providers
   d. All of the above are roles of a pharmacist

2. Which of the following is a responsibility of a pharmacist today (may select more than one)?(L-1-3)
   a. Accuracy of all prescription/medication orders processed
   b. Drug Utilization Evaluation
   c. Medication distribution
   d. All of the above

3. What is the primary role of a pharmacy technician today?(L-1-2)
   a. Assist the pharmacist
   b. Provide customer service
   c. Enter data
   d. Select the correct medication for a prescription

4. What type of duties does a pharmacy technician perform?(L-1-3)
   a. Judgmental
   b. Technical
   c. Both a and b
   d. Neither a nor b

5. Where should a pharmacy technician check for information on becoming a pharmacy technician in his or her state?(L-1-5)
   a. Food and Drug Administration
   b. National Association of Boards of Pharmacy
   c. State board of pharmacy
   d. United States Pharmacopoeia

6. Why is pharmacy technician certification important today in the practice of pharmacy?(L-1-5)
   a. Creates a minimum standard of care
   b. Provides the ability to work more effectively with pharmacists
   c. Provides greater patient care
   d. All of the above

7. Who regulates the practice of pharmacy in a state?(L-1-5)
   a. State DEA
   b. State EPA
   c. State FDA
   d. State board of pharmacy

8. Who is responsible for the work of a pharmacy technician in a pharmacy?(L-1-3)
   a. Lead pharmacy technician
   b. Pharmacist
   c. Pharmacist in charge
   d. Pharmacy technician trainer

9. Which of the following is *not* a characteristic of a pharmacy technician?(L-1-1)
   a. Caring
   b. Detail oriented
   c. Ethical
   d. Irresponsible

10. Which of the following is a characteristic of a pharmacy technician regardless of the setting?(L-1-1)
    a. Able to maintain confidential information
    b. Can work either alone or as part of a team
    c. Professional
    d. All of the above

11. Which of the following skills should a pharmacy technician possess?(L-1-1)
    a. Able to communicate effectively
    b. Able to work with a diverse group of people
    c. Strong keyboard skills
    d. All of the above

12. Which of the following knowledge skills should a pharmacy technician possess?(L-1-1)
    a. Able to interpret pharmacy abbreviations
    b. Able to perform pharmacy calculations
    c. Able to recognize the appropriate brand/generic names for a medication
    d. All of the above

13. Which of the following tasks may a pharmacy technician perform in a pharmacy?(L-1-3)
    a. Compound a prescription
    b. Input a patient's prescription into the computer
    c. Order medication for the pharmacy
    d. All of the above

14. Which of the following skills would be extremely beneficial in an institutional setting?(L-1-1)
    a. Hospital experience
    b. Knowledge and understanding of aseptic technique
    c. Strong understanding of automation, robotics, and computer technology
    d. All of the above

15. Which of the following skills would be helpful to possess if the technician is working in a long-term care facility?(L-1-7)
    a. Ability to repackage medications using various types of repackaging machinery
    b. Knowledge of dating methods used in repackaging medications
    c. Knowledge of labeling requirements for repackaging medications and records to be maintained
    d. All of the above

True/False

Mark True or False for each statement. If it is false, correct the statement to make it true.

1. _____ Pharmacy technicians do not need to have good math skills because 70% of the work performed is not math related.(L-1-1)

2. _____ An externship provides hands-on experience to individuals while they are studying to become pharmacy technicians.(L-1-6)

3. _____ The practice of pharmacy is highly respected among all other professions.(L-1-4)

4. _____ It is extremely important for pharmacy technicians to possess good communication skills, especially when they are counseling patients.(L-1-1)

5. _____ It is the responsibility of the pharmacist to oversee the work performed by pharmacy technicians.(L-1-3)

6. _____ The largest numbers of pharmacy technician positions are found in hospitals.(L-1-7)

7. _____ Certification is the process of demonstrating that an individual possesses the prerequisite skills for a profession.(L-1-5)

8. _____ Every state board of pharmacy requires that pharmacy technicians become certified before they begin their practice.(L-1-5)

9. _____ It is extremely important for pharmacy technicians to maintain a clean image.(L-1-1)

10. _____ In a retail pharmacy, pharmacy technicians prepare IVs for patients.(L-1-7)

Apply Your Knowledge

1. Why is there a need for pharmacy technicians today?(L-1-4)

_____

_____

2. Why do you want to become a pharmacy technician?(L-1-1)

_____

_____

3. Pretend that you are a pharmacist; what characteristics would you like to see in a pharmacy technician?(L-1-1)

_____

_____

4. What is the difference between certification and licensing?(L-1-5)

_____

_____

5. Why is it important for a pharmacy technician to be certified?(L-1-5)

_____

_____

6. What is the most important responsibility of a pharmacy technician?(L-1-3)

_____

_____

7. What is the importance of continuing education in the practice of pharmacy?(L-1-5)

_____

_____

8. A physician's office attempts to give you a new prescription for a patient over the telephone. What do you do?(L-1-3)

_____

_____

9. Which pharmacy setting do you find most interesting? Why?(L-1-7)

_____

_____

10. A patient who has hypertension asks you if he can take Drixoral; what do you tell the patient?(L-1-3)

_____

_____

Practice Your Knowledge

Materials Needed

1. Internet access to **www.ptcb.org**
2. Paper and pencil

Goal

To become familiar with the requirements for a pharmacy technician in your state.(L-1-5)

Assignment

Visit the PTCB Web site (**www.ptcb.org**) and find out if your state requires a pharmacy technician to be certified or to register with the board of pharmacy. Check to see if the states adjacent to your state require certification or registration. Then answer the following questions.(L-1-5).

Name of state?	
State board of pharmacy Web site?	
Registration required?	
Amount of registration fee?	
Length of registration?	
Certification required?	
If certification is required, which tests are accepted?	
Continuing education required? If yes, how many CEUs per registration period?	

Practice Your Knowledge

Materials Needed

1. Internet access
2. Paper and pencil

Goal

To become familiar with the various pharmacy technician careers in your community.[(L-1-7)]

Assignment

Using the Internet, identify the various career opportunities in your community and record the information in the following table.[(L-1-7)]

How many chain pharmacies are there and what are their names?	
How many independent pharmacies are there and what are their names?	
How many franchise pharmacies are there and what are their names?	
How many other retailers (grocery stores, mass merchandisers, and discounters) have a pharmacy in their store and what are their names?	
How many hospitals are in your community and what are their names?	
What are the names of the HMOs in your community?	
What are the names of any long-term care pharmacies in your community?	
What are the names of any home-infusion care pharmacies in your community?	
What are the names of any mail-order pharmacies in your community?	

Calculation Corner

A patient presents the following prescription to the pharmacy:

Dr. Andrew James
11608 Reynolds Ave.
Pittsburgh, PA 15219
412-344-1791

Mary Ellen   March 10, 2012
123 Triatholon Lane, Pittsburgh, PA 15217

Keflex 500 mg   #40
Take one capsule by mouth four times a day

Refill 0   Dr. Andrew James

1. How many days will the prescription last?   Work Out the Solution
    _____ (L-1-3)

Pharm Facts—Research

Complete Table 1-1 using either the
Physicians' Desk Reference or *Drug Facts and Comparisons*.(L-1-1)

Table 1-1

Brand Name	Generic Name	Strengths	Dosage Forms	List One Indications of the Medication	List Five Adverse Effects of the Medication
Achromycin					
Amoxil					
Augmentin					
Bactrim DS					
Biaxin					
Ceclor					
Ceftin					
Cipro					

(Continued)

Table 1-1 *(Continued)*

Brand Name	Generic Name	Strengths	Dosage Forms	List One Indications of the Medication	List Five Adverse Effects of the Medication
Cleocin					
Duracef					
E.E.S.					
Flagyl					
Floxin					
Gantrisin					
Garamycin					
Keflex					
Lorabid					
Macrodantin					
Minocin					
Pen Vee K					
Rocephin					
Vancocin					
Vantin					
Vibramycin					
Zithromax					

Did You Know?

Penicillin was accidentally discovered by Dr. Alexander Fleming at St. Mary's Hospital in London. He observed that a culture of *Staphylococcus aureus* had become contaminated by a species of *Penicillium* and that it was inhibiting bacterial growth.[L-1-1]

Basic Safety and Standards

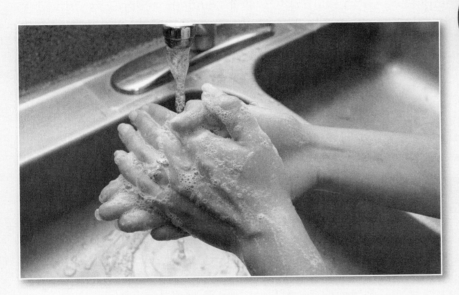

PTCB

In preparation for the certification examination, you should understand and perform activities associated with the following PTCB Knowledge Statements:

Domain I. Assisting the Pharmacist in Serving Patients

Knowledge of federal, state, and/or practice site regulations, codes of ethics, and standards related to the practice of pharmacy (1)

Domain II. Maintaining Medication and Inventory Control Systems

Knowledge of risk management opportunities (13)

Knowledge of policies, procedures, and practices regarding storage and handling of hazardous materials and wastes (22)

Learning Outcomes

Upon completion of this laboratory chapter, you will be able to:

L-2-1 Describe the role of regulatory agencies (CDC, OSHA) as they pertain to safety and standards in health care settings.

L-2-2 Define *infectious disease*, *nosocomial infections*, and *airborne* and *bloodborne diseases*.

L-2-3 List the four major types of nosocomial infections.

L-2-4 Describe methods to prevent airborne and bloodborne disease transmission.

L-2-5 Discuss the role of prevention in the spread of disease.

L-2-6 Discuss the role of hand hygiene in the prevention of disease.

L-2-7 Describe the proper technique for hand washing.

L-2-8 List and identify the proper use of personal protective equipment (PPE).

(Continued)

Learning Outcomes *(Cont'd)*

L-2-9 Define and explain the significance of policies and procedures as they pertain to documentation, reporting, and the prevention of disease transmission in health care organizations.

L-2-10 Describe the activities related to the incident report.

L-2-11 Describe HIV prophylaxis.

L-2-12 Discuss the importance of emergency preparedness (for example, first aid and CPR training).

L-2-13 Describe the proper handling, storage, and disposal of hazardous materials.

Domain III. Participating in the Administration and Management of Pharmacy Practice

Knowledge of storage and handling requirements for hazardous substances (13)

Knowledge of hazardous waste disposal requirements (14)

Knowledge of infection control policies and procedures (18)

Introduction to Basic Safety and Standards(L-2-1)

Full compliance with pharmacy policies and procedures is critical to maintain safety standards in any health care setting. In addition to state and federal laws, other agencies govern various areas of safety in various pharmacy environments—The Joint Commission (TJC; formerly JCAHO), for example. Such regulations represent the minimum standards to be met in any institution. Pharmacy technicians who function effectively in any health care facility must be aware of all of the regulations, standards, and policies in order to implement the appropriate procedure (action) for a specific situation.

Test Your Knowledge

Multiple Choice Questions

Answer the following multiple choice questions. When you have finished, check your answers and then review the areas where you need improvement.

1. Nosocomial refers to(L-2-2)
   a. an infection acquired in an inpatient setting.
   b. preventative measures to limit the spread of infection.
   c. an infection acquired in a community setting.
   d. application of personal protective equipment (PPE).

2. Bacteria that are *not* susceptible to multiple antibacterial agents demonstrate(L-2-2)
   a. multiple-drug allergenicity.
   b. multiple-drug sensitivity.
   c. multiple-drug resistance.
   d. multiple-pathogen resistance.

3. Which of the following is *not* a bloodborne pathogen?(L-2-4)
   a. Hepatitis B virus
   b. Human immunodeficiency virus
   c. Human papilloma virus
   d. Hepatitis C virus

4. Which of the following body fluids is generally *not* considered infectious unless it is contaminated with blood?(L-2-4, 2-5)
   a. Cerebrospinal fluid
   b. Saliva
   c. Semen
   d. Synovial fluid

5. The Centers for Disease Control and Prevention (CDC) recommends at least _____ antiretroviral agents for _____ weeks be used for HIV postexposure prophylaxis.(L-2-11)
   a. one, 2
   b. two, 3
   c. two, 4
   d. three, 5

6. Which of the following is true regarding HIV postexposure prophylaxis?(L-2-11)
   a. A prophylactic regimen should begin within hours of exposure.
   b. Immune globulin should be administered within 72 hours postexposure.

c. Hepatitis C vaccine should be administered to the patient within 24 hours of exposure.

d. Hepatitis B status of the source and infected persons must be evaluated.

7. Pharmacy technicians should follow standard precautions for[L-2-5]
   a. patients in ICU.
   b. patients in isolation.
   c. pediatric patients.
   d. all patients.

8. The difference in droplet transmission and airborne transmission of pathogens is[L-2-4, 2-5]
   a. the time of onset of illness.
   b. the size of the particles transmitted.
   c. the health care setting where the transmission occurred.
   d. none of the above.

9. Which of the following will *not* protect a pharmacy technician from contact transmission of pathogens?[L-2-5, 2-6, 2-7]
   a. Proper hand washing technique
   b. Holding his or her breath while in the same room with a patient
   c. Wearing gloves
   d. Wearing gowns or lab coats

10. Which of the following is not a component of hand hygiene?[L-2-6]
    a. Hand washing
    b. Antiseptic hand wash
    c. Gloveless hand shake
    d. Antiseptic hand rub

11. Which of the following is the proper term for bacteria impervious to multiple antibacterial agents?[L-2-2]
    a. Nosocomial infections
    b. Bloodborne pathogens
    c. Airborne pathogens
    d. Multidrug-resistant pathogens

12. Aseptic technique is employed to[L-2-4]
    a. increase productivity.
    b. maintain product sterility.
    c. decrease processing time.
    d. none of the above.

13. _____ is an organization that is primarily concerned with the control and prevention of disease.[L-2-1]
    a. FDA
    b. CDC

c. DEA
d. OSHA

14. _____ is an organization primarily concerned with workplace safety.[L-2-1]
    a. DEA
    b. TJC
    c. OSHA
    d. CDC

15. Which of the following is *not* a food borne pathogen?[L-2-2]
    a. Shigella
    b. Salmonella
    c. Smallpox
    d. Botulism

16. The _____ is a written document that facilitates and organizes employer and employee actions during workplace emergencies.[L-2-9, 2-11]
    a. EAP
    b. EPA
    c. DEA
    d. FDA

17. A list of potential workplace fire hazards, types of fire control devices, and fire protection equipment are contained in the[L-2-9]
    a. EAP.
    b. FPP.
    c. OSHA.
    d. none of the above.

18. Which of the following is *not* a biologic agent associated with bioterrorism?[L-2-4, 2-5]
    a. Ricin
    b. Smallpox
    c. Anthrax
    d. Triclosan

19. All of the following can contribute to pharmacy technician exposure to hazardous substances except[L-2-13]
    a. not using recommended biological safety cabinets.
    b. using appropriate personal protective equipment.
    c. hazardous handling practices.
    d. improper practices in drug preparation areas.

20. Which of the following is *not* appropriate for the preparation of hazardous drugs?[L-2-13]
    a. Class II biologic safety cabinet
    b. Class III biologic safety cabinet
    c. Type B biologic safety cabinet
    d. Horizontal biologic safety cabinet

21. Which of the following does *not* increase the risk for exposure while using a biologic safety cabinet (BSC)?[L-2-13]
    a. Using a poor BSC cleaning technique
    b. Allowing clutter and unnecessary items in the BSC
    c. Wearing two pairs of gloves while working in the BSC
    d. Blocking the BSC vent

22. TJC recommends that the Pharmacy Infection Control Policies and Procedures address all of the following except[L-2-1]
    a. storage of nonsterile products.
    b. irrigation solution preparation.
    c. preparation of parenteral nutrition products.
    d. infection surveillance, prevention, and control.

23. Which of the following is *not* a component of HIV postexposure prophylaxis?[L-2-11]
    a. Retrovir (zidovudine)
    b. Zovirax (acyclovir)
    c. Epivir (lamivudine)
    d. Videx (didanosine)

24. Hazardous drug-related wastes should be disposed of according to _____ standards for hazardous waste disposal.[L-2-13]
    a. EAP
    b. EPA
    c. FPP
    d. DEA

True/False

Mark True or False for each statement. If it is false, correct the statement to make it true.

1. _____ The use of gloves eliminates the need for hand washing.[L-2-6]

2. _____ A nosocomial infection is one that is acquired at home or while in the community.[L-2-2]

3. _____ Wearing surgical masks may help reduce the spread of airborne diseases.[L-2-5, 2-8]

4. _____ To avoid needlestick injuries, needles should not be recapped or broken.[L-2-4, 2-5]

5. _____ Synovial fluid is considered potentially infectious only if it contains blood.[L-2-3, 2-5]

6. _____ *Pseudomonas aeruginosa* is a pathogen that is associated with nosocomial infections.[L-2-2]

7. _____ An antiseptic agent is a substance that, when applied to the skin, causes a reduction in the number of microbial flora.[L-2-4, 2-5]

8. _____ Pharmacy technicians who perform sterile compounding must wear gloves, hair covers, gowns, and shoe covers.[L-2-8]

9. _____ The pharmacy technician is not responsible for assisting the pharmacist in controlling and preventing infection in the pharmacy.[L-2-5, 2-9]

10. _____ According to OSHA standards, employers must retain only an Emergency Action Plan.[L-2-1, 2-9]

11. _____ Used needles and syringes should be disposed of in a sharps container.[L-2-4, 2-9]

Apply Your Knowledge

1. List five biologic agents that may be employed in bioterrorist events.(L-2-2)

   _____

   _____

   _____

2. Identify the method of internal reporting in the event of a workplace accident or injury. Provide examples of situations where external reporting would be required.(L-2-1, 2-9)

   _____

   _____

   _____

3. ASHP defines hazardous substances as those that can exhibit at least one of the following effects on humans and/or animals.(L-2-1, 2-9)

   _____

   _____

   _____

4. List five ways the pharmacy technician can aid in the proper storage of hazardous materials.(L-2-9, 2-13)

   _____

   _____

   _____

5. Identify five drugs that should be handled as hazardous substances.(L-2-13)

   _____

   _____

   _____

Practice Your Knowledge

Materials Needed

1. Sink
2. Warm running water
3. Liquid antibacterial soap
4. Low-lint disposable towels

Goal

To be able to demonstrate proper hand washing technique and hand hygiene.(L-2-6)

Assignment

1. Wet hands with warm running water.(L-2-6)
2. Apply soap and thoroughly distribute over hands.(L-2-6)
3. Vigorously rub hands together for 10 to 15 seconds, generating friction on all surfaces of the hands and fingers, including the backs of the hands, backs of fingers, and under the fingernails.(L-2-6)
4. Rinse hands completely to remove all traces of soap, especially between fingers.
5. Dry hands using dry paper towels.(L-2-6)
6. Use a paper towel to turn off the faucet in the event that there are no foot controls.(L-2-6)

Practice the task until you are able to obtain a fair or excellent self-evaluation, then obtain a final evaluation from your instructor.

Evaluation Form

	Self-Evaluation			Instructor Evaluation		
Task	**Rating**			**Rating**		
Basic Hand Washing	**Excellent**	**Fair**	**Poor**	**Excellent**	**Fair**	**Poor**
Wet hand with warm running water						
Apply and distribute soap thoroughly.						
Vigorously rub hands including: - palms of hands - backs of hands - between fingers - under fingernails						
Rinse hands removing all traces of soap.						
Dry hand using a paper towel.						
Avoid contamination of hands by using a paper towel to turn off faucet or open the door.						

Calculation Corner

You have received an order for amoxicillin suspension 150 mg every 8 hours for 10 days. The pharmacy stocks amoxicillin 125 mg/5 mL.

1. How many milliliters will be required for each dose? _____ (L-2-6, 2-7)
2. What is the minimum amount of amoxicillin needed for the prescription? _____ (L-2-6, 2-7)

Work Out the Solution

Pharm Facts—Research

Accutane (tretinoin) is a medication that was identified in the chapter as a hazardous substance.

Using reference materials, research this agent with respect to its therapeutic use, adverse drug reactions, why it is considered hazardous, and how it is packaged. Be prepared to discuss your findings with your classmates.[L-2-1]

Did You Know?

According to the Department of Labor, Occupational Safety and Health Administration (OSHA), over 30 million American workers are exposed to hazardous chemicals in their workplaces. OSHA's Hazard Communication Standard (HCS) is intended to ensure that these workers and their employers are informed of the identities of these hazardous chemicals, associated health and safety hazards, and appropriate protective measures. The HCS covers some 650,000 hazardous chemical products found in over 3 million establishments.[L-2-1]

Communication and Customer Service

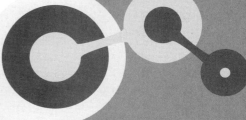

3

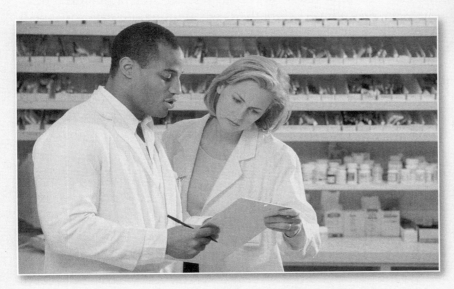

PTCB

In preparation for the certification examination, you should understand and perform activities associated with the following PTCB Knowledge Statements:

Domain I. Assisting the Pharmacist in Serving Patients

Knowledge of customer service principles (71)

Knowledge of communication techniques (72)

Knowledge of confidentiality requirements (73)

Domain II. Maintaining Medication and Inventory Control Systems

Knowledge of the written, oral, and electronic communication channels necessary to ensure appropriate follow-up and problem resolution (24)

Learning Outcomes

Upon completion of this laboratory chapter, you will be able to:

L-3-1 Identify and explain the components of the communication process.

L-3-2 Differentiate between the various types of communication used in pharmacy.

L-3-3 Identify various forms of nonverbal communication.

L-3-4 Explain the importance of effective communication in the practice of pharmacy.

L-3-5 Explain the results that may occur due to poor communication in the practice of pharmacy.

L-3-6 Identify various solutions to communication problems in a pharmacy.

L-3-7 Explain the meaning of customer service in the practice of pharmacy.

(Continued)

Learning Outcomes *(Cont'd)*

L-3-8   Define and identify the customer in the practice of pharmacy.

L-3-9   Identify the tools used to provide outstanding customer service.

L-3-10   Explain the need for patient privacy and confidentiality in the practice of pharmacy.

Domain III. Participation in the Administration and Management of Pharmacy Practice

> Knowledge of lines of communication throughout the organization (2)
>
> Knowledge of written, oral, and electronic communications (5)

Introduction to Communication and Customer Service(L-3-2)

Every prescription or medication order processed in a pharmacy requires communication between members of the physician's office, the pharmacy, and the patient. The pharmacist and pharmacy technician communicate using both verbal and nonverbal methods when filling prescriptions/medication orders. Communication is required whenever collecting information from or counseling the patient. The pharmacy staff's effectiveness as communicators plays a significant role in the quality of care provided to customers and the service they receive at the pharmacy.

Test Your Knowledge

Multiple Choice Questions

Answer the following multiple choice questions. When you have finished, check your answers and then review those areas that need improvement.

1. Which of the following directions may demonstrate the flow of communication in a pharmacy?(L-3-2)
   a. Downward
   b. Lateral
   c. Upward
   d. All of the above

2. Which of the following is a physical barrier in a pharmacy?(L-3-6)
   a. A husband who is dropping off a prescription for his wife and will not allow her to answer questions needed to complete her patient profile. The female patient is capable of speaking fluent English.
   b. A long line of customers are waiting for their prescription.
   c. The height of the pharmacy counter.
   d. Using pharmacy terminology to a patient who is experiencing difficulty in speaking English.

3. Which of the following is an example of positive communication (may select more than one)?(L-3-6)
   a. Looking at the customer
   b. Smiling at the customer
   c. Speaking to the customer in terms he or she will understand
   d. All of the above

4. Which of the following is an example of active listening (may select more than one)?(L-3-1)
   a. Asking questions
   b. Listening for feelings
   c. Paraphrasing
   d. All of the above

5. Which of the following is *not* an example of good telephone etiquette?(L-3-9)
   a. Answering the telephone promptly
   b. Collecting information from the customer
   c. Interrupting the patient
   d. Providing accurate and complete information to the customer

6. Which of the following factors does *not* affect the interpretation of nonverbal communication?(L-3-6)
   a. Cultural factors
   b. Factors affecting the ability to speak and understand English
   c. Psychological factors
   d. Social factors

7. Which of the following methods of communication involves body movement and facial expression?(L-3-3)
   a. Kinesics
   b. Oculesics
   c. Proxemics
   d. None of the above

8. Which type of distance is used when collecting information from a customer?(L-3-3)
   a. Intimate
   b. Personal
   c. Public
   d. Social

9. Which of the following reactions may occur when a customer find a prescription error has occurred?(L-3-9)
   a. Anger
   b. Anxiety
   c. Confusion
   d. All of the above

10. Which of the following is *not* a stage of the dying process?(L-3-9)
    a. Acceptance
    b. Bargaining
    c. Denial
    d. Resentment

11. What type of problems may arise from continual stress?(L-3-9)
    a. Emotional
    b. Mental
    c. Physical
    d. All of the above

12. Which of the following is *not* an example of an external customer?(L-3-8)
    a. Human resource department of your employer
    b. Nurse
    c. Patient
    d. Physicians

13. Which organization accredits continuing education for pharmacists and pharmacy technicians?(L-3-9)
    a. ACPE
    b. APHA
    c. ASHP
    d. PTCB

14. What is the minimum passing score for continuing education for a pharmacy technician?(L-3-9)
    a. 55%
    b. 60%
    c. 65%
    d. 70%

15. Which of the following is *not* a barrier in communication with a customer?(L-3-6)
    a. Shyness
    b. The height of the pharmacy counter
    c. Time
    d. All of the above

True/False

Mark True or False for each statement. If it is false, correct the statement to make it true.

1. _____ Playing music in the pharmacy may be a barrier for communication.(L-3-6, 3-9)

2. _____ A pharmacy technician should always use words the customer can understand.(L-3-4, 3-6)

3. _____ Asking the customer questions is a good way to see he or she understands the pharmacist's instructions.(L-3-6)

4. _____ Listening is a passive process.(L-3-1)

5. _____ If a pharmacy technician is actively listening to the customer, he or she may develop empathy toward the customer.(L-3-6, 3-9)

6. _____ Empathy and sympathy have the same meaning.(L-3-6, 3-9)

7. _____ The telephone can be used to receive a new prescription for a patient from a

physician's office, as a way for a patient to call in a refill prescription, or as a way to obtain a refill prescription for a patient.(L-3-9)

8. _____ Culture is learned.(L-3-7)

9. _____ Patient inserts may be used in counseling patients.(L-3-3, 3-9)

10. _____ All patient information is to remain confidential.(L-3-10)

11. _____ Eustress is positive stress.(L-3-9)

12. _____ Positive attitudes improve customer service.(L-3-9)

13. _____ An individual's work ethic is affected by events during his or her childhood and adolescence.(L-3-6)

14. _____ Professionals obtain satisfaction through their work.(L-3-9)

15. _____ Understanding a patient's illness improves customer service.(L-3-9)

Matching(L-3-3)

Match the body language with the behavior.

_____ 1. Holding arms crossed on chest

_____ 2. Biting fingernails

_____ 3. Looking downward

_____ 4. Standing with hands on hips

_____ 5. Rubbing hands

_____ 6. Tapping fingers

_____ 7. Tilting head

_____ 8. Tugging at ear

_____ 9. Walking erectly

_____ 10. Walking with hands in pockets

A. Confidence

B. Disbelief

C. Anticipation

D. Dejection

E. Indecision

F. Defensiveness

G. Impatience

H. Readiness, aggression

I. Insecurity, nervousness

J. Interest

Apply Your Knowledge

1. Ms. Dowd brings in her prescription bottle for a refill of Fosamax on a Saturday afternoon. There are no refills remaining on the prescription. Despite numerous attempts to contact her physician, the pharmacy was unable to do so.(L-3-9)

   a. What is the problem?

   _____

   b. What are possible solutions to this problem?

   _____

2. Mr. Kunze calls the pharmacy on Monday to refill a prescription. He informs the pharmacy technician that no refills remain on the prescription and that his physician is expecting a call from the pharmacy to approve the refill. Mr. Kunze provides the pharmacy technician with his home, office, and cell telephone numbers. He informs the technician that he will pick up the prescription after 4 P.M. on Wednesday. Wednesday afternoon at 5:15 P.M., Mr. Kunze arrives at the pharmacy to pick up the prescription. The pharmacy

technician searches for the prescription for 5 minutes and finally informs Mr. Kunze that they have not been able to obtain permission to refill his prescription for Lipitor. Mr. Kunze becomes extremely upset.[L-3-6, 3-9]

a. Does Mr. Kunze have a reason to be upset with the pharmacy? Why or why not?

_____

b. What could the pharmacy have done to prevent this incident from occurring?

_____

c. How would you handle the solution?

_____

d. Evaluate how the pharmacy technician handled the situation.

_____

3. It is Monday morning and Mr. Dagit presents a new prescription for hypertension to the pharmacy. The pharmacy technician examines the prescription and asks the pharmacist if they stock this medication. The pharmacist informs the technician they do not have the medication in stock.[L-3-9]

a. What are some possible solutions to this problem?

_____

_____

b. What would you say to Mr. Dagit?

_____

_____

c. Evaluate how the pharmacy technician handled the situation.

_____

_____

4. How does the appearance of the pharmacy affect the communication process between the pharmacy team and the customer? Use examples in your discussion.[L-3-3, 3-9]

_____

_____

5. Ms. Vargas brings in a new prescription to be filled at your pharmacy. Her new prescription does not have her address, birth date, or home telephone listed on it. You attempt to obtain this information from the patient and realize that she does not understand or speak English. You enter her name in the pharmacy computer to determine if she has ever filled a prescription at your pharmacy.
After several attempts, you conclude that she has never filled a prescription at your pharmacy. How would you collect the following information from the patient: home address, birth date, home telephone number, medication allergies, and insurance information?[L-3-6, 3-9]

_____

_____

6. Which of the following types of barriers (environmental, personal, patient, or time) provides the greatest obstacle to the pharmacy customer? Give examples with your explanation.[L-3-6]

_____

_____

7. Identify the five most important work habits of a pharmacy technician. Why did you select them?[L-3-9]

_____

_____

8. Is a pharmacy technician a professional? Why or why not?[L-3-9]

_____

_____

9. Mary Locke has been a customer of your pharmacy for several years. Recently, she has been extremely angry and irritable when she has visited the pharmacy. Today, you notice that her hair appears to be thinning and she has lost weight. She informs you she has been diagnosed with both ovarian and uterine cancer. She is undergoing chemotherapy. How do you react? What do you say to her?[L-3-6, 3-9, 3-10]

_____

_____

10. Using the drugs listed in the Pharm Facts—Research section of this chapter, explain how the pharmacist might instruct a patient who does not speak English how to take a medication.[L-3-9]

_____

_____

Practice Your Knowledge

Materials Needed

1. Paper
2. Pencil

Goal

To observe and interpret the body language of the pharmacy staff.

Assignment

Visit your local pharmacy and observe the body language of both the pharmacist and the pharmacy technician(s). List examples of body language demonstrated by the pharmacy team in the following table.[L-3-3]

Describe the clothing the pharmacist was wearing.	
Describe the clothing the pharmacy technician was wearing.	
Were the pharmacy staff members wearing name tags?	
Did they acknowledge you when you approached the pharmacy counter? How long did it take them to acknowledge you?	
Did they smile at you?	
Describe their facial expressions.	
Did they look you in the eye?	
Were they standing up straight or were they slouching?	
Describe their hand motions.	
If you asked them a question, did they move toward you?	
Describe the appearance of the pharmacy.	
How would you describe their attitude toward their customers? Why?	
Did the phone ring while you were standing there? If so, how many times did it ring before it was answered?	
Did their body language create a positive or negative impression? Why?	

Practice Your Knowledge

Materials Needed

1. Pencil
2. Written prescription

Goal

To collect a patient's information to prepare a patient profile from a "difficult" patient.

Assignment

Select two students to participate in a role-playing situation, where one student plays the role of the pharmacy technician and the other student portrays a patient dropping off a new prescription. The pharmacy technician attempts to gather information and the patient (considered to be difficult) has difficulty answering the questions. The pharmacy technician asks the following questions: [L-3-6]

What is the patient's name, address, and telephone number?	
Has the patient filled a prescription before at this pharmacy?	
What is the patient's birth date?	
Does the patient have a prescription drug card? If so, what prescription drug coverage does he or she have?	
Is the patient allergic to any medications?	
Does the patient have any other allergies?	
Is the patient taking any other prescription medications? If so, which ones?	
Does the patient take any over-the-counter medications or herbal supplements? If so, which ones?	
Does the patient want a generic medication if one is available?	
Does the patient want the medication in a child-resistant container?	

Calculation Corner

A patient has been instructed to inject 35 units of Humulin 70/30 insulin subcutaneously once a day.

1. How many milliliters would the patient need to draw up in the syringe with each injection?[L-3-6]

Work Out the Solution

Pharm Facts—Research

Using a *Physicians' Desk Reference* or *Drug Facts and Comparisons*, complete Table 3-1.

Table 3-1

Brand Name	Generic Name	Strengths	Indications	Contraindications	Adverse Effects
Anusol HC Suppositories					
Bactrim Pediatric Suspension					
Cortisporin Otic Suspension					

(Continued)

Table 3-1 *(Continued)*

Brand Name	Generic Name	Strengths	Indications	Contraindications	Adverse Effects
Domeboro Tablets					
EES Chewable Tablets					
Epi-Pen					
Epsom Salts					
Fleet Enema					
Flonase					
Humulin 70/30 Insulin					
Keflex Capsules					
Lotrimin Cream					
Metamucil					
Monistat 7 Vaginal Cream					
Mycelex Troche					
Nitrostat					
Nizoral Shampoo					
Ocean Nasal Spray					
St. Joseph's Chewable Aspirin					
Tessalon Perles					
Timoptic Ophthalmic Drops					
Tylenol Pediatric Drops					
Zovirax Ointment					

Did You Know?

Many pharmacies have software to allow them to print prescription labels and handouts in Spanish for their Hispanic customers. Some pharmacies have software that will print prescription labels in Braille for customers who are visually impaired.[L-3-4]

Ethics, Law, and Regulatory Agencies

REGISTRANTS INVENTORY OF DRUGS SURRENDERED

OMB Approval No. 1117-0007

U.S. Department of Justice / Drug Enforcement Administration

PACKAGE NO.

The following schedule is an inventory of controlled substances which is hereby surrendered to you for proper disposition.

FROM: *(include Name, Street, City, State and ZIP Code in space provided below.)*

Signature of applicant or authorized agent

Registrant's DEA Number

Registrant's Telephone Number

NOTE: CERTIFIED MAIL (Return Receipt Requested) IS REQUIRED FOR SHIPMENTS OF DRUGS VIA U.S. POSTAL SERVICE. See instructions on reverse (page 2) of form.

NAME OF DRUGS OR PREPARATION	Number of Containers	CONTENTS (Number of grams, tablets; ounces or other units per container)	Controlled Substance Content, (Each unit)	FOR DEA USE ONLY		
				DISPOSITION	QUANTITY	
					GMS.	MGS.
Registrants will fill in Columns 1,2,3 and 4 ONLY.						
1	2	3	4	5	6	7

Learning Outcomes

Upon completion of this laboratory chapter, you will be able to:

L-4-1 Explain *ethics*.

L-4-2 Identify the ethical conduct required of pharmacy technicians.

L-4-3 Explain the importance of the following pharmacy legislation:

a. Pure Food and Drug Act; Sherley Amendment; Harrison Narcotic Act; Food, Drug and Cosmetic Act

b. Durham-Humphrey Act; Kefauver-Harris Act

c. Controlled Substance Act; Poison Prevention Packaging Act

d. Occupational Safety and Health Act; Drug Listing Act; Medical Device Amendments

(Continued)

PTCB

In preparation for the certification examination, you should understand and perform activities associated with the following PTCB Knowledge Statements:

Domain I. Assisting the Pharmacist in Serving Patients

Knowledge of federal, state, and/or practice site regulations, code of ethics, and standards pertaining to the practice of pharmacy (1)

Knowledge of pharmaceutical, medical, and legal developments that affect the practice of pharmacy (2)

Knowledge of state-specific prescription transfer regulations (3)

Knowledge of information to be obtained from patient /patient's representative (21)

Knowledge of required prescription order refill information (22)

Knowledge of formula to verify the validity of a prescriber's DEA number (23)

Learning Outcomes *(Cont'd)*

e. Orphan Drug Act; Drug Price Competition and Patent Term Restoration Act; Prescription Drug Marketing Act; Omnibus Budget Reconciliation Act of 1987

f. Omnibus Budget Reconciliation Act of 1990; Dietary Supplement Health and Education Act of 1994

g. Health Insurance Portability and Accountability Act of 1996; Comprehensive Methamphetamine Control Act; FDA Modernization Act

h. Medicare Modernization Act; USP <797>; Anabolic Steroid Control Act

i. Isotretinoin Safety and Risk Management Act

L-4-4 Relate the meaning of *schedule* to the Controlled Substance Act of 1970 and the criteria for placing a medication in a particular schedule.

L-4-5 Differentiate between an initial inventory, biennial inventory, and perpetual inventory as they relate to pharmacy.

L-4-6 Describe the methods of filing prescription and pharmacy records.

L-4-7 Explain the requirements issued by the CMS for Medicaid Tamper Resistant prescription pads.

L-4-8 Identify the following regulatory agencies and their role in the practice of pharmacy:

  a. Food and Drug Administration (FDA); Drug Enforcement Administration (DEA)

  b. Occupational Safety and Health Administration (OSHA); Centers for Medicare and Medicaid Services (CMS) and The Joint Commission (TJC) (formerly The Joint Commission Accreditation of Healthcare Organizations, JCAHO)

L-4-9 Identify the role of the state board of pharmacy in each state and the National Association of Boards of Pharmacy.

L-4-10 Explain *law*.

L-4-11 Differentiate between federal law, state law, and torts.

L-4-12 Explain *respondeat superior*.

Knowledge of techniques for detecting forged or altered prescriptions (24)

Knowledge of National Drug Code (NDC) components (34)

Knowledge of special directions and precautions for patient/patient's representative regarding preparation and use of medications (39)

Knowledge of requirements for mailing a prescription (42)

Knowledge of requirements for dispensing controlled substances (44)

Knowledge of record-keeping requirements for medication dispensing (46)

Knowledge of documentation requirements for controlled substances, investigational drugs, and hazardous waste (68)

Knowledge of confidentiality requirements (73)

Domain II. Maintaining Medication and Inventory Control Systems

Knowledge of drug product laws and regulations and professional standards related to obtaining medication supplies, durable medical equipment, and products (4)

Knowledge of the use of DEA Controlled substance ordering forms (9)

Knowledge of legal and regulatory requirements and professional standards for preparing, labeling, dispensing, distributing, and administering medications (18)

Knowledge of medication distribution and control systems requirements for controlled substances, investigational drugs, and hazardous materials and wastes (23)

Domain III. Participation in the Administration and Management of Pharmacy Practice

Knowledge of State Board of Pharmacy regulations (11)

Knowledge of the Americans with Disabilities Act requirements (25)

Knowledge of security procedures related to data integrity, security, and confidentiality (26)

Knowledge of legal requirements regarding archiving (30)

Introduction to Ethics, Law, and Regulatory Agencies(L-4-9)

The practice of pharmacy is regulated by both federal and state laws and pharmacy regulations enacted by the State Board of Pharmacy. A pharmacy technician needs to be aware of these laws and regulations. Failure to follow them may lead to a reprimand, suspension of the right to practice as a pharmacy technician, a fine issued by the state board of pharmacy, or even legal consequences resulting in a fine and/or jail sentence, especially where controlled substances are involved.

Test Your Knowledge

Multiple Choice Questions

Answer the following multiple choice questions. When you have finished, check your answers and then review those areas that need improvement.

1. An NDC number indicates(L-4-3d)
   a. manufacturer and drug.
   b. drug and package size.
   c. manufacturer, drug, and package size.
   d. manufacturer, drug, and cost.

2. The Poison Prevention Act of 1970 provided(L-4-3c)
   a. ipecac should be readily available to the public for accidental poisonings.
   b. established conditions for drugs that should not be in a child-resistant container.
   c. pharmacists should be trained in first aid and accidental poisonings.
   d. none of the above.

3. OBRA-90(L-4-3f)
   a. mandated Drug Utilization Evaluation.
   b. mandated that in each community there is a pharmacist on duty or on call 24 hours a day.
   c. mandated that pharmacists distribute drug literature with all prescriptions.
   d. mandated that pharmacists provide educational programs to the public.

4. The Drug Price Competition and Patent Term Restoration Act of 1984 encouraged(L-4-3e)
   a. the development of generic drugs and new drug products.
   b. the creation of orphan drugs.
   c. the creation of investigational drugs.
   d. the elimination of outdated drugs.

5. Which of the following is *not* an exemption from using child-resistant containers?(L-4-3c)
   a. A single time dispensing of a product in a noncompliant container as ordered by a physician
   b. A single time or blanket dispensing of a product in a noncompliant container as requested by the patient or customer in a signed statement

c. Drugs dispensed to institutional patients, provided that they are to be dispensed by employees of the institution

d. All of the above are exemptions

6. Which of the following does *not* need to be packaged in child-resistant containers?(L-4-3c)
   a. Sublingual nitroglycerin tablets
   b. Oral contraceptives
   c. Inhalation aerosols
   d. All of the above

7. What was the purpose of the Orphan Drug Act of 1983?(L-4-3e)
   a. To develop pharmaceutical products that have no medical use in the world
   b. To develop pharmaceutical products with a limited use by providing manufacturers tax incentives and exclusive licenses
   c. To encourage the creation and innovation of new drugs by streamlining the process for generic drug approval and by extending the patent licenses
   d. To provide drug utilization review for each patient

8. What does the Prescription Drug Marketing Act of 1987 prohibit?(L-4-3e)
   a. The reimportation of drugs into the United States except by the drug manufacturer
   b. The sale or trading of drug samples
   c. The distribution of samples other than to individuals who are licensed to prescribe them
   d. All of the above

9. Under OBRA-90, patients must receive(L-4-3f)
   a. Drug Utilization Evaluation.
   b. an offer to counsel.
   c. an offer for medication delivery if they are unable to pick them up.
   d. all of the above.
   e. a and b only.

10. Which of the following is an example of Drug Utilization Evaluation?(L-4-3f)
    a. Screening of potential drug therapy problems due to therapeutic duplication
    b. Drug disease contraindications
    c. Drug-drug interactions
    d. All of the above

11. Which of the following would be considered an example(s) of counseling under OBRA-90?(L-4-3f)
    a. Providing the name and description of the medication
    b. Providing special directions and precautions for preparation, administration, and use by the patient
    c. Providing common side effects of a medication to a patient
    d. All of the above

12. What will occur if a pharmacy fails to adhere to OBRA-90?(L-4-3f)
    a. Revocation of the the pharmacy's permit
    b. Revocation of the DEA number
    c. Loss of Medicaid participation
    d. Fine by the FDA

13. Which of the following is *not* true concerning the filling of Accutane prescriptions?(L-4-3i)
    a. The quantity prescribed can't exceed a 30-day supply.
    b. The prescription must be filled within 7 days of the prescription being written.
    c. Original prescriptions must be hand written.
    d. Refilled prescriptions may be called in to the pharmacy.

14. Which of the following is *not* true concerning the filling of Accutane prescriptions?(L-4-3i)
    a. Women must undergo two negative pregnancy tests prior to receiving their initial prescription.
    b. Women must commit to simultaneously use two effective birth control methods for one month prior, during, and after cessation of taking Accutane.
    c. Women must sign a patient information/consent form about Accutane and birth defects, as well as a consent form about other potential serious risks.
    d. Women must undergo a pregnancy test.

15. What is the purpose of HIPAA?(L-4-3g)
    a. To develop uniform health care procedures for the health care profession
    b. To provide comprehensive privacy for all patients in the United States
    c. To develop equitable compensation for all health care providers
    d. To provide educational materials to the public concerning public health care issues

16. Which federal agency is responsible for recalling drugs?[(L-4-8a)]
    a. FDA
    b. DEA
    c. NAPB
    d. State Boards of Pharmacy

17. Which federal agency is responsible for placing a drug in a particular schedule?[(L-4-8a)]
    a. FDA
    b. DEA
    c. NAPB
    d. State Boards of Pharmacy

18. Which organization is responsible for the practice of pharmacy in a particular state?[(L-4-9)]
    a. FDA
    b. DEA
    c. NAPB
    d. State Boards of Pharmacy

19. Which organization is responsible for the accreditation of hospitals, home health care agencies, and long-term care pharmacies?[(L-4-8b)]
    a. CMS
    b. FDA
    c. TJC
    d. NABP

20. Which law prevents drug supplement manufacturers from issuing disease claims?[(L-4-3f)]
    a. FDCA 1938
    b. Orphan Drug Act of 1983
    c. Prescription Drug Marketing Act of 1987
    d. DSHEA 1994

21. Which law prohibits the sale or distribution of pharmaceutical samples to anyone other than those licensed to prescribe them?[(L-4-3e)]
    a. FDCA 1938
    b. Durham-Humphrey Amendment
    c. Prescription Drug Marketing Act of 1987
    d. FDA Modernization Act

22. Which of the following is the federal legend?[(L-4-3b)]
    a. Federal law prohibits dispensing without a prescription.
    b. Federal law prohibits the dispensing of this medication to anyone other than intended by prescription.
    c. Federal law prohibits dispensing of medication without a child-resistant container.
    d. Federal law prohibits providing information to anyone other than the intended patient.

23. Which of the following would *not* be a correct DEA number for Dr. Wilfred Opakunle?[(L-4-3c)]
    a. AO1234563
    b. BO5555555
    c. MO2468139
    d. WO1234563

24. What was the intent of the Pure Food and Drug Act of 1906?[(L-4-3a)]
    a. To ensure that all food and drugs were pure
    b. To ensure that all food and drugs were pure and safe
    c. To ensure that all food and drugs were pure, safe, and effective
    d. To prohibit the interstate transportation or sale of adulterated and misbranded food and drugs

25. What was the intent of the Kefauver-Harris Amendment?[(L-4-3b)]
    a. To ensure that all food and drugs were pure
    b. To ensure that all food and drugs were pure and safe
    c. To ensure that all food and drugs were pure, safe, and effective
    d. To prohibit the interstate transportation or sale of adulterated and misbranded food and drugs

26. What is the difference between a prescription medication and an over-the-counter medication?[(L-4-3b)]
    a. Cost
    b. Indications or uses
    c. Physician's supervision
    d. Side effects

27. What form is used to report a theft of controlled substances to the authorities?[(L-4-3c)]
    a. DEA Form 41
    b. DEA Form 106
    c. DEA Form 222
    d. DEA Form 363

28. What form is used to transfer Schedule II medications between pharmacies?[(L-4-3c)]
    a. DEA Form 41
    b. DEA Form 106
    c. DEA Form 222
    d. DEA Form 363

29. Which type of inventory shows the amount of medication on hand in a pharmacy at a particular time?(L-4-3c)
    a. Biannual inventory
    b. Biennial inventory
    c. Initial Inventory
    d. Perpetual inventory

30. Which schedule of medications may be partially filled for up to 60 days from the date of issuance for long-term care facility patients or terminally ill patients?(L-4-3c)
    a. Schedule II
    b. Schedule III
    c. Schedule IV
    d. Schedule V

31. Under what schedule does an "exempt narcotic" fall?(L-4-3c)
    a. Schedule II
    b. Schedule III
    c. Schedule IV
    d. Schedule V

32. What is the maximum number of bottles of an exempt narcotic can be purchased in 48 hours?(L-4-3c)
    a. 1
    b. 2
    c. 3
    d. 4

33. How old must one be to purchase an exempt narcotic?(L-4-3c)
    a. 16
    b. 18
    c. 21
    d. 65

34. Which form is used to destroy all controlled substances?(L-4-3c)
    a. DEA Form 10
    b. DEA Form 41
    c. DEA Form 222
    d. DEA Form 363
    e. None of the above

35. How many schedules were created under the Controlled Substance Act?(L-4-3c)
    a. 1
    b. 2
    c. 3
    d. 4
    e. 5

36. How is it determined in which schedule a controlled substance is placed?(L-4-3c)
    a. Cost
    b. Approved medical use in United States
    c. Potential for abuse
    d. Side effects
    e. b and c only

37. What is the maximum number of different Schedule II drugs that can be ordered at one time on a single DEA Form 222?(L-4-3c)
    a. 1
    b. 5
    c. 10
    d. No limit

38. If an error is made ordering Schedule II drugs, what must be done?(L-4-3c)
    a. Correct the error on the form by initialing it.
    b. Throw away the form.
    c. File the form with the DEA.
    d. Place the form in the pharmacy safe and retain it. Use a new order form and write the order.

39. Who may write prescriptions for controlled substances?(L-4-3c)
    a. A doctor
    b. A medical doctor
    c. A medical doctor with a DEA number
    d. None of the above

40. If an "emergency prescription" for a Schedule II medication is called in to the pharmacy, when must the pharmacy receive a handwritten prescription from the prescriber?(L-4-3c)
    a. 24 hours
    b. 48 hours
    c. 1 week
    d. 30 days

41. Which schedule includes heroin?(L-4-3c)
    a. I
    b. II
    c. III
    d. IV
    e. V

42. How many refills authorized by a physician are allowed for Schedule II drugs?(L-4-3c)
    a. 0
    b. 1
    c. 2
    d. 3
    e. 4
    f. 5

43. How many refills authorized by a physician are allowed for Schedule III drugs?[(L-4-3c)]
    a. 0
    b. 1
    c. 2
    d. 3
    e. 4
    f. 5

44. Which law created the FDA?[(L-4-3a)]
    a. Ethics
    b. Pure Food and Drug Act of 1906
    c. FDCA 1938
    d. Durham-Humphrey 1951

45. Which law is being violated if a medication is not labeled properly?[(L-4-3a)]
    a. Ethics
    b. Pure Food and Drug Act of 1906
    c. FDCA 1938
    d. Durham-Humphrey 1951

46. What is being violated if a pharmacy technician fails to remain competent in the practice of pharmacy?[(L-4-2)]
    a. Ethics
    b. Pure Food and Drug Act of 1906
    c. FDCA 1938
    d. Durham-Humphrey 1951

47. Which law is being violated if a medication is dispensed in a dirty container?[(L-4-3a)]
    a. Ethics
    b. Pure Food and Drug Act of 1906
    c. FDCA 1938
    d. Durham-Humphrey 1951

48. Which of the following is being broken if a pharmacy technician tells his or her spouse that a celebrity is taking Drug X?[(L-4-2)]
    a. Ethics
    b. Pure Food and Drug Act of 1906
    c. FDCA 1938
    d. Durham-Humphrey 1951

49. Which law prohibited the interstate transportation of adulterated and misbranded medications?[(L-4-3a)]
    a. Ethics
    b. Pure Food and Drug Act of 1906
    c. FDCA 1938
    d. Durham-Humphrey 1951

50. Which law required the submission of NDA to the FDA?[(L-4-3a)]
    a. Ethics
    b. Pure Food and Drug Act of 1906
    c. FDCA 1938
    d. Durham-Humphrey 1951

51. Which of the following is being violated if pharmacy technician fails to ensure the health and safety of patients?[(L-4-2)]
    a. Ethics
    b. Pure Food and Drug Act of 1906
    c. FDCA 1938
    d. Durham-Humphrey 1951

52. How many refills authorized by a physician are allowed for Schedule IV drugs?[(L-4-3c)]
    a. 0
    b. 1
    c. 2
    d. 3
    e. 4
    f. 5

53. How may a patient receive a Schedule III drug from a doctor?[(L-4-3c)]
    a. Written prescription
    b. Telephoned prescription
    c. Faxed prescription
    d. All of the above

54. When refilling Schedules III–V drugs, during what period must it be completed before the prescription becomes void?[(L-4-3c)]
    a. 1 month from the date the prescription was written
    b. 3 months from the date the prescription was written
    c. 6 months from the date the prescription was written
    d. 12 months from the date the prescription was written
    e. No time period

55. Which of the following is true considering partial filling of Schedules III–V drugs?[(L-4-3c)]
    a. Each partial filling is recorded in a similar manner as a refilling.
    b. The total quantity dispensed in partial fillings does not exceed the total quantity prescribed.
    c. No partial fillings may occur after 6 months of the date the prescription was written.
    d. All of the above.

Acronyms

Print the meaning of the following acronyms.(L-4-3a, 4-3f, 4-8a, and 4-8b)

CMS _____

DEA _____

FDA _____

DUE _____

EPA _____

HIPAA _____

INDA _____

TJC _____

NABP _____

NDA _____

NDC _____

OSHA _____

Apply Your Knowledge

1. A patient drops off a prescription for 60 tablets of Valium 5 mg with five refills indicated on it. The patient requests that the prescription be transferred to another pharmacy. What must you do and when?(L-4-3c)

    _____

    _____

2. A patient brings in a prescription for 30 tablets of Vicodin with 0 refills. The patient has money for only 15 tablets. What do you tell the patient regarding this request?(L-4-3c)

    _____

    _____

3. A prescription is called in to the pharmacy for a patient and you notice on the patient's profile that he or she has requested e-z open packaging. What should you do?(L-4-3c)

    _____

    _____

4. A patient presents a prescription for 100 tablets of Ritalin 5 mg on Monday afternoon. You notice that you have only 50 tablets and your daily delivery from your wholesaler has already arrived. What can you do?(L-4-3c)

    _____

    _____

5. You are processing a prescription for a patient and you notice that it is contraindicated with other medications the patient is taking. What should you do?(L-4-3f)

    _____

    _____

6. The pharmacist is away from the pharmacy for a brief time. A friend's mother enters the pharmacy and asks to purchase a 4-ounce bottle of Robitussin AC. According to the "exempt narcotics register" you notice that the patient purchased a bottle 72 hours ago. What do you do and why?(L-4-3c)

    _____

    _____

7. The pharmacist is talking on the phone to a physician when a patient comes to the pharmacy counter and asks you to recommend an OTC medication for a specific condition. In the past, you have heard the pharmacist recommend Product X for the very same condition. What do you do and why?(L-4-3f)

    _____

    _____

8. A patient is picking up a prescription at the pharmacy and you are aware that his wife has a filled prescription awaiting her. Should you inform the patient of this situation? Why or why not?(L-4-2)

    _____

    _____

9. Explain the three methods of filing prescriptions and maintaining prescription records in a pharmacy.(L-4-3c, 4-6)

    _____

    _____

10. Heroin is classified as a Schedule I controlled substance. Why is it classified as a Schedule I medication?(L-4-3c)

    _____

    _____

Practice Your Knowledge

Materials Needed

1. *Drug Facts and Comparisons* or
2. *Physicians' Desk Reference*

Goal

To identify problems that may occur when receiving prescriptions for controlled substances and what corrective actions should be taken by pharmacy staff.[L-4-3c]

Assignment

In the following table, list the problem and solution for each prescription written.[L-4-3]

1.

Dr. Andrew James 111 Brandon Way, Suite 300 Washington, DC 20007 202-687-0100

Jerry Dagit 300 Craft Ave., Apt. 6	January 3, 2010 Pittsburgh, PA 15209
Percocet #30 I tab po q 4–6 hr prn pain	
Refill × 1	Dr. Andrew Shedlock

2.

Dr. Brandon Mizner 111 Brandon Way, Suite 102 Washington, DC 20007 FM1234563

Joe Kunze	January 4, 2010
Ambien CR 6.25 mg #30 One po q hs prn sleep	
Ref × 6	Dr. Brandon Mizner

3.

Dr. Mary Ellen 111 Brandon Hill Way, Suite 208 Reston, VA 20194-1215 BE1234563

Randy Kraisinger
Xanax   0.5 mg   #100
Ref × 6

4.

```
                          Dr. Ken Yarhi
                   1100 Wilson Blvd., Suite 310
                      Washington, DC 20007
                         202-687-2000
                          FY1111111

Mickey Kirkpatrick                      January 6, 2010
1100 Arlington Blvd., Arlington, VA 22207

Oxycontin 40 mg
I tab po qd

Refill one time                         Dr. Yarhi
```

Prescription #	Problem	Solution
1.		
2.		
3.		
4.		

Practice Your Knowledge

Materials Needed

1. Internet
2. Pencil

Goal

To become familiar with the recent actions imposed by your State Board of Pharmacy on both pharmacists and pharmacy technicians.[L-4-9]

Assignment

Using the Internet as a source of information, visit your State Board of Pharmacy Web site and view the 10 most recent actions taken by the board against either pharmacists or pharmacy technicians. Record them in the following table.[L-4-9]

Individual	Brief Description of the Incident	Board of Pharmacy Action	What Can Be Learned from This Situation?

Calculation Corner

Calculate the last number in each of the
following numbers to make them valid DEA
numbers.[L-4-3c]

AS012347 _____

BC222333 _____

FD765432 _____

MM122159 _____

AZ346702 _____

Pharm Facts—Research

Complete the table 4-1 using either the *Physicians'
Desk Reference* or *Drug Facts and Comparisons*.[L-4-3c]

Table 4-1

Brand Name	Generic Name	Strengths	Schedule	List Two Indications of the Medication	List Three Adverse Effects of the Medication
Ativan					
Dalmane					
Darvocet N 100					
Darvon 65					
Demerol					
Dilaudid					
Donnagel PG					
Fiorcet					
Fiorinal					
Halcion					
Librium					
Lortab					
Oxycontin					
Parepectolin					
Percocet					
Percodan					
Restoril					
Ritalin					
Robitussin AC					
Stadol NS					

(Continued)

Table 4-1   *(Continued)*

Brand Name	Generic Name	Strengths	Schedule	List Two Indications of the Medication	List Three Adverse Effects of the Medication
Terpin Hydrate with Codeine					
Tranxene					
Tussionex					
Tylenol with Codeine					
Tylox					
Valium					
Vicodin					
Vicoprofen					
Xanax					

Did You Know?

A pharmacist, pharmacy technician, or other health care professional can be suspended or even terminated from his or her position for violating HIPAA regulations in an institution regardless of the health care setting.[L-4-3g]

Pharmacology and Medications

Unit 2

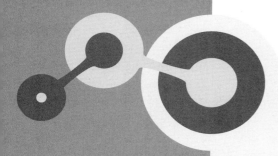

5 Measurements and Calculations

Learning Outcomes

Upon completion of this laboratory chapter, you will be able to:

L-5-1 Convert roman numerals to the equivalent Arabic number.

L-5-2 Multiply and divide fractions.

L-5-3 Convert fractions to decimals, ratios, and percents.

L-5-4 Convert numbers to percents.

L-5-5 Distinguish between various metric prefixes used in the practice of pharmacy.

L-5-6 Convert units between the metric, apothecary, avoirdupois, and household systems.

L-5-7 Convert temperatures between Celsius and Fahrenheit.

L-5-8 Convert time between the 12-hour and 24-hour clocks.

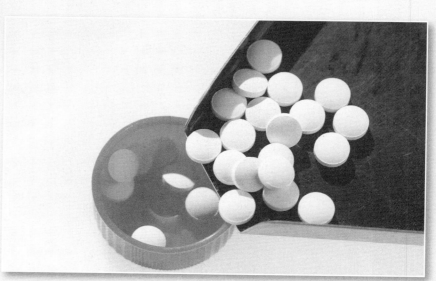

PTCB

In preparation for the certification examination, you should understand and perform activities associated with the following PTCB Knowledge Statement:

Domain I. Assisting the Pharmacist in Serving Patients

Knowledge of pharmaceutical and medical abbreviations and terminology (4)

Knowledge of generic and brand names of pharmaceuticals (5)

Knowledge of pharmacy calculations (50)

Knowledge of measurement systems (51)

Learning Outcomes *(Cont'd)*

L-5-9   Interpret a written drug order.

L-5-10   Calculate the day's supply of a medication prescribed by a physician.

L-5-11   Identify on a drug label the drug name, form, dosage strength, route, manufacturer, and storage information.

L-5-12   Indicate the appropriate equipment for measuring the appropriate quantity of solids and liquids in the practice of pharmacy.

L-5-13   Convert the dosage ordered to the desired dose.

L-5-14   Convert the desired dose to the amount to administer.

L-5-15   Calculate the appropriate dose for a patient based upon his or her age, weight, or body surface area.

L-5-16   Calculate the amount of drug of a given concentration to prepare a prescription yielding different concentrations.

L-5-17   Calculate the ending concentration of a preparation after diluting it with a diluent.

L-5-18   Calculate the correct quantities to be used in preparing a solution or semisolid using alligation.

L-5-19   Calculate the flow rate of an intravenous fluid.

L-5-20   Calculate the correct drop factor to be used for an intravenous solution.

L-5-21   Calculate the number of drops per minute a patient will receive when given the flow rate and drop factor.

L-5-22   Explain the importance of calculations in the practice of pharmacy.

L-5-23   Demonstrate an understanding and application of proportions in pharmacy calculations.

L-5-24   Use dimensional analysis in performing pharmacy calculations.

L-5-25   Demonstrate an understanding of the application of international units and milliequivalents in pharmacy.

L-5-26   Interpret a prescription or medication order.

L-5-27   Reduce or enlarge a formula to meet the requirements of either a prescription or medication order.

L-5-28   Demonstrate an understanding of specific gravity and its application in compounding a product.

Introduction to Measurements and Calculations (L-5-22)

Calculations are a crucial part of a pharmacy technician's responsibility. Each day the technician performs many calculations, and each must be done accurately. Fortunately, by learning and practicing a few basic mathematical procedures, you can develop the skills necessary to perform these tasks with confidence. This chapter of the laboratory applications manual focuses on practicing these skills.

Test Your Knowledge

Multiple Choice Questions

Answer the following multiple choice questions. When you have finished, check your answers and then review those areas that need improvement.

1. Which of the following fractions is equivalent to 3/5?(L-5-3)
   a. 2/3
   b. 9/12
   c. 12/20
   d. 12/15

2. Which of the following fractions is equivalent to 7/8?(L-5-3)
   a. 14/15
   b. 14/16
   c. 15/24
   d. 21/32

3. The fraction 3/8 is equal to _____(L-5-3)
   a. 0.375.
   b. 0.215.
   c. 0.35.
   d. 0.45.

4. The fraction 2/15 is equal to approximately _____(L-5-3)
   a. 0.215.
   b. 0.113.
   c. 0.125.
   d. 0.133.

5. The fraction 2/5 is equal to _____(L-5-3)
   a. 40%.
   b. 35%.
   c. 30%.
   d. 25%.

6. The fraction 5/12 is equal to approximately _____(L-5-3)
   a. 35.65%.
   b. 41.67%.
   c. 45.23%.
   d. 51.20%.

7. 1/3 × 2/5 =(L-5-2)
   a. 2/15
   b. 2/8
   c. 3/8
   d. 5/12

8. 3/4 × 1/2 =(L-5-2)
   a. 4/6
   b. 3/6
   c. 3/8
   d. 1/4

9. 2/3 ÷ 4/5 =(L-5-2)
   a. 4/15
   b. 5/6
   c. 3/8
   d. 3/4

10. 1.5 tsp =(L-5-6)
    a. 2.5 mL
    b. 5 mL
    c. 7.5 mL
    d. 10 mL

11. 60 mL =(L-5-6)
    a. 2 tbsp
    b. 4 tbsp
    c. 6 tbsp
    d. 8 tbsp

12. 75 mL =(L-5-6)
    a. 4 fl oz
    b. 3.5 fl oz
    c. 3 fl oz
    d. 2.5 fl oz

13. 2.5 L =(L-5-6)
    a. 25 mL
    b. 250 mL
    c. 2500 mL
    d. 25,000 mL

14. 230 g =(L-5-6)
    a. 0.23 kg
    b. 2.3 kg
    c. 23,000 kg
    d. 230,000 kg

15. 28°C =(L-5-7)
    a. −2.2°F
    b. 14.0°F
    c. 82.4°F
    d. 93.6°F

16. 55°F =(L-5-7)
    a. 12.7°C
    b. 48.3°C
    c. 50°C
    d. 67°C

17. Dosage ordered: Lopressor 25 mg Dose on hand: Lopressor 50-mg tablets; calculate the amount to administer.(L-5-14)
    a. 0.5 tablet
    b. 1 tablet
    c. 1.5 tablets
    d. 2 tablets

18. Dosage ordered: Diuril 0.5 g
    Dose on hand: Diuril 250-mg tablets; calculate the amount to administer.(L-5-6 and L-5-14)
    a. 0.5 tablet
    b. 1 tablet
    c. 1.5 tablets
    d. 2 tablets

19. Dosage ordered: morphine sulfate 0.25 g
    Dose on hand: morphine sulfate 30 mg/mL;
    calculate the amount to administer.(L-5-6 and L-5-14)
    a. 0.5 mL
    b. 1 mL
    c. 1.5 mL
    d. 2 mL

20. Dosage ordered: Dilantin 225 mg
    Dose on hand: Dilantin 125 mg/5mL;
    calculate the amount to administer.(L-5-14)
    a. 5 mL
    b. 7 mL
    c. 9 mL
    d. 11 mL

21. Dosage ordered: Vistaril 75 mg
    Dose on hand: Vistaril 25 mg/5mL;
    calculate the amount to administer.(L-5-14)
    a. 1.5 tsp
    b. 2 tsp
    c. 2.5 tsp
    d. 3 tsp

22. Dosage ordered: Dilaudid 0.8 mg
    Dose on hand: Dilaudid 2 mg/mL;
    calculate the amount to administer.(L-5-14)
    a. 0.2 mL
    b. 0.4 mL
    c. 0.6 mL
    d. 0.8 mL

23. Dosage ordered: Thorazine 40 mg
    Dose on hand: Thorazine 25 mg/mL;
    calculate the amount to administer.(L-5-14)
    a. 0.6 mL
    b. 0.8 mL
    c. 1.2 mL
    d. 1.6 mL

24. According to Clark's Rule, if the adult dose of
    a medication is 250 mg, the dose for a 45-lb
    child would be _____(L-5-15)
    a. 50 mg.
    b. 75 mg.
    c. 100 mg.
    d. 150 mg.

25. According to Clark's Rule, if the adult dose
    of a medication is 75 mg, the dose for a 60-lb
    child would be _____(L-5-15)
    a. 30 mg.
    b. 40 mg.
    c. 50 mg.
    d. 60 mg.

26. According to Clark's Rule, if the adult dose of
    a medication is 200 mg, the dose for a 75 lb
    child would be _____(L-5-15)
    a. 160 mg.
    b. 120 mg.
    c. 140 mg.
    d. 100 mg.

27. According to Young's Rule, if the adult dose of
    a medication is 150 mg, the dose for an 8-year-
    old child would be _____(L-5-15)
    a. 50 mg.
    b. 55 mg.
    c. 60 mg.
    d. 65 mg.

28. According to Young's Rule, if the adult dose of
    a medication is 50 mg, the dose for a 5-year-
    old child would be approximately_____(L-5-15)
    a. 15 mg.
    b. 20 mg.
    c. 20 mg.
    d. 25 mg.

29. In order to prepare 100 mL of a 2.5% solution
    from a 10% solution, you would need _____(L-5-16)
    a. 20 mL of the 10% solution.
    b. 25 mL of the 10% solution.
    c. 30 mL of the 10% solution.
    d. 35 mL of the 10% solution.

30. In order to prepare 500 mL of a 1.2% solution
    from a 30% solution, you would need _____(L-5-16)
    a. 20 mL of the 30% solution.
    b. 25 mL of the 30% solution.
    c. 30 mL of the 30% solution.
    d. 35 mL of the 30% solution.

31. In order to prepare 450 mL of a 6% solution
    from a 1% and a 10% solution, you would
    need _____ mL of the 1% solution and _____ mL
    of the 10% solution. (L-5-18)
    a. 250 mL of 1% + 200 mL of 10%
    b. 175 mL of 1% + 275 mL of 10%
    c. 200 mL of 1% + 250 mL of 10%
    d. 150 mL of 1% + 300 mL of 10%

32. In order to prepare 100 mL of a 1.5% solution
    from a 1% and a 3% solution, you would need
    _____ mL of the 1% solution and _____ mL of
    the 3% solution. (L-5-18)
    a. 25 mL of 1% + 75 mL of 3%
    b. 40 mL of 1% + 60 mL of 3%
    c. 60 mL of 1% + 40 mL of 3%
    d. 75 mL of 1% + 25 mL of 3%

33. What is the flow rate for 1000 mL infused over 8 hours?[(L-5-19)]
    a. 100 mL/h
    b. 125 mL/h
    c. 150 mL/h
    d. 175 mL/h

34. What is the flow rate for 500 mL infused over 6 hours?[(L-5-19)]
    a. 102 mL/h
    b. 96 mL/h
    c. 83 mL/h
    d. 71 mL/h

35. What is the flow rate for 1800 mL infused over 12 hours?[(L-5-19)]
    a. 100 mL/h
    b. 125 mL/h
    c. 150 mL/h
    d. 175 mL/h

36. What is the flow rate for 250 mL infused over 30 minutes via 15 gtts/mL tubing?[(L-5-5.21)]
    a. 75 gtts/min
    b. 125 gtts/min
    c. 150 gtts/min
    d. 175 gtts/min

37. What is the flow rate for 0.5 L infused over 6 hours via 15 gtts/mL tubing?[(L-5-21)]
    a. 21 gtts/min
    b. 24 gtts/min
    c. 28 gtts/min
    d. 32 gtts/min

38. What is the flow rate for 1000 mL infused over 10 hours via microdrip tubing?[(L-5-21)]
    a. 40 gtts/min
    b. 60 gtts/min

    c. 80 gtts/min
    d. 100 gtts/min

39. A physician orders an IV to be infused at 30 mg/h for 24 hours. What is the total gram dose for the patient?[(L-5-23)]
    a. 0.72 mg
    b. 0.72 g
    c. 720 mg
    d. 720 g

40. What is the flow rate for 1800 mL infused over 12 hours via 10 gtts/mL tubing?[(L-5-21)]
    a. 15 gtts/min
    b. 20 gtts/min
    c. 25 gtts/min
    d. 30 gtts/min

41. Complete the following chart using the household system of measurements to demonstrate their equivalence to other household measurements.[(L-5-6)]

mL	tsp	tbsp	fl oz	cup	pt	qt	gal
							1
						1	
					1		
				1			
960							
	96						
		48					
			16				
				8			
					10		
						8	
							2

Apply Your Knowledge

Using the math skills and formulas introduced in this chapter; solve the following problems.

1. The physician orders sodium bicarbonate, gr XXX.[(L-5-1, 5-6)]
   If the unit dose on hand is 0.3 g tablets, how many tablets are needed for the doses ordered? _____

2. A pediatric product is formulated to contain 100 mg of erythromycin ethylsuccinate in each dropper (2.5 mL) of the product.[(L-5-6, 5-23)]
   How many grams of ethylsuccinate would be required to prepare 100 bottles each containing 50 mL of the preparation?
   _____

3. A pharmacy receives the following prescription:[(L-5-27)]

Salicylic Acid	1%
Menthol	1/4%
Triamcinolone Cream	0.1%

   How much salicylic acid and menthol should be used to prepare 1 lb of this compound? _____

4. If a patient were to receive 5 mg/kg of a drug, how much would a 132-lb patient need?[(L-5-6, and L-5-15)]
   _____

5. How many gallons of Coca-Cola fountain syrup are needed to package 144 4-oz bottles?(L-5-6, 5-23)

   _____

6. The dose for vincristine based on the patient's body weight is 25 mcg/kg. The drug is available as 500 mcg/mL. The patient weighs 165 lb.(L-5-6 and L-5-15)
   How many milliliters are used for each dose?

   _____

7. A physician writes an order for a 52-lb child for 400,000 units/kg/day. Each dose is administered in a 50-mL bag of D5W IVPB. The drug is available as 500,000 units per mL.(L-5-6, L-5-15, L-5-23 and L-5-25.)
   How many milliliters will be used in each IVPB?

   _____

8. A 20% solution has been diluted to 400 mL and is now a 5% solution.(L-5-16)
   What was the beginning volume of the 20% volume? _____

9. You have a container in which you are keeping one cup of a substance with a specific gravity of 1.25. You add a cup of different liquid with a specific gravity of 0.93.(L-5-28)
   What does the content of the container now weigh? _____

10. You need to prepare 60 mL of 0.025% solution.(L-5-16)
    How many milligrams of powder will you need to dissolve? _____

11. You are asked to weigh out 10 g of menthol and told to dissolve in distilled water to make a 5% solution. An order is received from a physician and you are asked to make a 2.5% solution from the 5% solution.(L-5-17)
    What will be the final volume?

    _____

12. You are asked to prepare 125 mL of a 1:8 Nystatin suspension and you have in stock a 1:6 solution.(L-5-16)
    How many milliliters of the 1:6 solution will you need? _____

13. You are asked to prepare 30 mL of a 1:4 acetic acid solution and you have in stock a 2:5 solution.(L-5-16)
    How many milliliters of the 2:5 solution will you use? _____

14. A 14% (w/v) topical solution is available in the pharmacy. The pharmacist receives an order for 1 L of a 1:4000 solution.(L-5-3, 5-16)
    How much of the original solution will be necessary to fill the order? _____

15. You are asked to prepare 280 mL of 1:5 Nitroprusside solution, and you have in stock a 30% solution.(L-5-3 and L-5-16)
    How many milliliters of the 30% solution will you use? _____

16. You are given 120 mL of a 50% (w/v) potassium chloride solution and are told to add 300 mL of sterile water to it.(L-5-17)
    What will be the final (w/v) percentage concentration of the solution be? _____

17. The pharmacist has weighed out 10 g of coal tar and given it to you with the instructions to compound a 1% ointment.(L-5-17)
    What will be the final weight of the correctly compounded prescription? _____

18. If 500 mL contains 0.5 g of drug, what is the percentage strength? _____ (L-5-3, 5-17)

19. You make a 5% hydrocortisone ointment by using 25% hydrocortisone and generic ointment base.(L-5-17)
    How much of the ointment base must you add to make a total of 500 g? _____

20. You are asked to make 120 mL of 3% NaCl solution. Using the 5% NaCl stock solution and distilled water, how much do you use? (L-5-17)

    _____

21. You have a 65% solution and a 25% solution available. You are asked to make a 40% solution.(L-5-18)
    How many milliliters of the 65% solution and 25% solution will be needed to make 100 mL of the 40% solution? _____

22. You have a 10% ointment and a 1% ointment available. You are asked to make a 2% ointment.(L-5-18)
    How many grams of the 10% and 1% ointment will be needed to make 45 g of a 2% ointment?

    _____

23. How many milliliters of a 1:200 iodine solution and a 7.5% iodine solution are needed to make 100 mL of a 3.5% solution? (L-5-3 and L-5-18)

    _____

24. A prescription is written for Allopurinal liquid 20 mg/mL in Ora-Plus: Ora-Sweet 1:1 (label with a shelf life of 60 days).(L-5-3 and L-5-18)
    How many tablets of allopurinal 100 mg are needed to prepare 150 mL? _____

25. You are preparing hydrocortisone 2.4 g in 240 mL of Lubriderm lotion.(L-5-3,)
    What percentage strength should appear on the label of the container? _____

26. Human albumin 75 mL is to be given at the rate of 15 mL/h. Assuming an administration set with a DF of 15 was used,(L-5-19, 5-21)
    a. How long in hours will it take to run the infusion? _____
    b. What is the flow rate in drops per minute? _____

27. 10,000 units of heparin in 500 mL NS is administered to a patient at the rate of 80 units/min.
    What is the rate of infusion in drops per minute if the administration set used is calibrated at 15 gtts/mL? _____ (L-5-21)

28. A request is sent to the pharmacy by a nurse for a large-volume parenteral solution to be infused at the rate of 100 mL for 24 hours.(L-5-10)
    How many 1-L bags will the pharmacy supply? _____

29. If 1 L of D10W is started at 1500 hr on Wednesday, at what time and day will the next liter bag be started if the infusion rate is 100 mL/hour? _____ (L-5-8, 5-19)

30. A doctor has prescribed drug A for a patient to be infused at the rate of 5 g/h. Drug A is available in the pharmacy as a 12% w/v IV solution packaged in 500-mL bottles.(L-5-19,5-23)
    What will be the rate of infusion in milliliters per hour and how long will a 500-mL bottle last? _____

31. What quantity of IVF in milliliters will a patient receive if the infusion rate was set at 50 mL/h, was started at 1100 hr and stopped at 2100 hr? _____ (L-5-8, 5-19)

32. How much volume will be delivered if a patient receives 5% dextrose at 60 mL/h for 96 hours? Express your answer in liters. _____ (L-5-6. 5-23)

33. 1000 mL is to be administered at 20 gtts/min using a 15-drop set.
    What is the flow rate in milliliters per hour? _____ (L-5-19)

34. 1-Liter D5NS is to be infused at the rate of 66 gtts/min for 5 hours.
    What will be the drop factor of the IV set selected? _____ (L-5-20)

35. 45 mEq of potassium chloride is to be given in 500-mL IVF at a rate of 125 mL/h.
    How many milliequivalents per hour will the patient receive? _____ (L-5-25)

Practice Your Knowledge

Materials Needed

1. Calculator
2. Nomogram

Goal

To compare the results of the various methods used for calculating pediatric dosages.(L-5-15)

Assignment

An 11-year-old male child weighing 95 lb and is 62 in. tall is prescribed cephalexin where the adult dose is 500 mg qid.

Calculate the dose for this child using Young's Rule, Clark's Rule, and body surface area. Which method of calculation is the best for this child and why?(L-5-15)

Calculation Corner

From the following formula, calculate the quantity of each ingredient required to make 240 mL of calamine lotion.(L-5-27)

Calamine 80 g
Zinc Oxide 80 g
Glycerin 20 g
Bentonite Magma 250 mL
Calcium Hydroxide Sol qs 1000 mL

How much of each ingredient will you need to prepare this compound?(L-5-27)

Work Out the Solution

Pharm Facts—Research

Using *Drug Facts and Comparisons* or the *Physicians' Desk Reference,* complete Table 5-1. Calculate the number of grams of active ingredient in each container by using the concepts learned in this chapter. [L-5-3, 5-6]

Table 5-1

Brand Name	Generic Name	Number of Grams of Active Ingredient in Container	Indication	List Three Contraindications	List Five Adverse Effects
Norvir 80 mg/mL 240 mL					
Protopic 0.1% 60 g					
Atrovent Nasal Spray 0.03% 15 mL					
Augmentin 400 mg–57 mg/ 5 mL 100 mL					
Bactroban 2% Ointment 22 g					
Flonase Nasal Spray 50 mcg/ spray 120 metered sprays					
Paxil Oral Suspension 10 mg/5 mL 250 mL					
Finacea Gel 15% 15 g					
Astelin Nasal Spray 137 mcg/ inh 200 metered sprays					
Elocon Cream 0.1% 45 g					
Neoral Oral Solution 100 mg/mL 50 mL					
Mentax 1% 15 g					
Risperdal 1 mg/mL 30 mL					
Zofran Oral Solution 4 mg/ 5 mL 50 mL					
Ziagen Oral Solution 20 mg/ mL 240 mL					
Retrovir Syrup 50 mg/5 mL 240 mL					
Zantac 15 mg/mL 1 pint					
Soltamox 10 mg/5 mL 150 mL					
Alphagen P 0.15% 15 mL					
Restasis 0.05% 32 × 0.4 mL vials					

Did You Know?

The metric system is the official system for weights and measures according to the USP–NF. The apothecary system was at one time considered the traditional system of measurement in the practice of pharmacy. Although certain components of this system are still used, the avoirdupois system of measurement is used primarily along with the metric system in commerce today.[L-5-6]

Introduction to Pharmacology

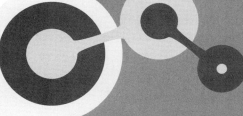

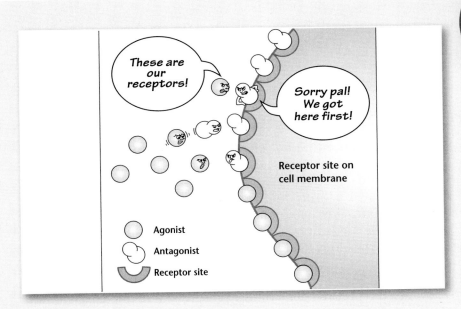

PTCB

In preparation for the certification examination, you should understand and perform activities associated with the following PTCB Knowledge Statements:

Domain I. Assisting the Pharmacist in Serving Patients

Knowledge of therapeutic equivalence (6)

Knowledge of drug interactions (12)

Knowledge of effects of patient's age (14)

Knowledge of pharmacology (16)

Knowledge of common and severe side effects or adverse effects, allergies, and therapeutic contraindications associated with medications (17)

Knowledge of drug indications (18)

Knowledge of drug stability (52)

Domain II. Maintaining Medication and Inventory Control Systems

Knowledge of bioavailability standards (8)

Learning Outcomes

Upon completion of this laboratory chapter, you will be able to:

L-6-1 Differentiate between the following terms: *pharmacology, pharmacokinetics, pharmacy,* and *toxicology.*

L-6-2 Discuss the principles affecting pharmacokinetics.

L-6-3 Explain the processes (absorption, distribution, metabolism, and elimination) involved in pharmacokinetics.

L-6-4 Explain the factors affecting the absorption of a drug.

L-6-5 Explain the issues affecting the distribution of a drug in the body.

L-6-6 Explain the factors affecting the metabolism of a drug in the body.

L-6-7 Explain the factors affecting the elimination of a drug in the body.

(Continued)

Introduction to Pharmacology(L-6-1)

Pharmacology is a science that deals with the knowledge of the source of a drug; the physical and chemical properties of a drug; the biochemical and physiological effects of a drug; the mechanisms of action of a drug; the therapeutic use of a drug; and the pharmacokinetics involving the drug. Every day pharmacy technicians assist pharmacists in processing prescriptions and/or medication orders. Pharmacy technicians use their knowledge of pharmacology during the Drug Utilization Evaluation phase of prescription processing, which improves patient outcomes. Various situations involving the usage of medications and a knowledge of pharmacology allows the pharmacy technician to provide better service to the patient.

Test Your Knowledge

Multiple Choice Questions

Answer the following multiple choice questions. When you have finished, check your answers and then review those areas that need improvement.

1. Which of the following may affect the absorption of a medication?(L-6-4)
   a. Patient's age
   b. Patient's health
   c. Presence of food in the digestive tract
   d. All of the above

2. Which of the following organs are involved with the elimination of a drug from the body?(L-6-7)
   a. Kidneys
   b. Lungs
   c. Skin
   d. All of the above

3. With respect to bioavailability, which of the following is true?[(L-6-15)]
   a. A common method by which generic firms show bioequivalence is by measuring "bioavailability."
   b. Bioavailability is defined by federal regulations as the rate and extent to which the active ingredient or active moiety is absorbed from a drug product and becomes available at the site of action.
   c. From a pharmacokinetic point of view, bioavailability data provide an estimate of the relative fraction of the administered drug that is absorbed into the systemic circulation.
   d. All of the above are true.

4. Who assigns a nonproprietary name to a drug?[(L-6-16)]
   a. DEA
   b. Drug manufacturer
   c. FDA
   d. USP

5. Which of the following factors affect the absorption of a drug in the body?[(L-6-4)]
   a. Drug concentration
   b. Drug solubility
   c. Route of administration
   d. All of the above

6. Where does a drug accumulate in the body?[(L-6-3)]
   a. Fat
   b. Extracellular reservoirs
   c. Plasma proteins
   d. All of the above

7. Which of the following processes use non-microsomal enzymes in the metabolism of a drug?[(L-6-3, 6-6)]
   a. Conjugation
   b. Hydrolysis
   c. Oxidation
   d. All of the above

8. Which of the following processes is *not* part of the elimination of a drug?[(L-6-3, 6-7)]
   a. Active tubular secretion
   b. Glomerular filtration
   c. Passive glomerular filtration
   d. Passive tubular reabsorption

9. Which of the following physiochemical factors affect drug transfer across a membrane?[(L-6-3)]
   a. Cell membrane
   b. Electrolytes and pH
   c. Passive transport
   d. All of the above

10. Which of the following does *not* affect the absorption of a drug?[(L-6-3, 6-4)]
    a. Absorbing surface area
    b. Circulation to the absorption site
    c. Drug concentration
    d. Homeostasis

11. Which of the following terms meets chemical and physical standards established by government or regulatory agencies?[(L-6-15)]
    a. Bioavailability equivalent
    b. Biologically equivalent
    c. Chemically equivalent
    d. Therapeutically equivalent

12. Which of the following therapeutic equivalent codes have undergone in vivo or in vitro data supporting bioequivalence?[(L-6-15)]
    a. AA
    b. AB
    c. AN
    d. AO

13. Which of the following therapeutic equivalence codes indicates that the drug requires additional FDA investigation?[(L-6-15)]
    a. B*
    b. BB
    c. BC
    d. BD

14. Which type of drug distribution requires that a drug go from a higher to a lower concentration?[(L-6-4)]
    a. Active transport (diffusion)
    b. Filtration
    c. Passive transport (diffusion)
    d. Redistribution

15. Which of the following is defined as the study and identification of natural products used as drugs?[(L-6-17)]
    a. Pharmacognosy
    b. Pharmacology
    c. Pharmacodynamics
    d. Pharmacokinetics

16. Which of the following is *not* true about pharmacology?(L-6-1)
    a. Pharmacology is a science that deals with the physical and chemical properties of a drug.
    b. Pharmacology is a science that deals with the compounding of a drug.
    c. Pharmacology is a science that deals with the therapeutic use of a drug.
    d. Pharmacology is a science that deals with the dosage form of a drug.

17. Which of the following drug interactions results when a drug blocks the effects of a drug?(L-6-17)
    a. Additive effects
    b. Antagonism
    c. Potentiation
    d. Synergism

18. Which of the following pregnancy categories is awarded to a drug for which studies have not been performed in pregnant women or in which animal studies have not demonstrated fetal risk?(L-6-20)
    a. Pregnancy Category A
    b. Pregnancy Category B
    c. Pregnancy Category C
    d. Pregnancy Category NR

19. Which of the following is *not* true regarding drug use in geriatric patients?(L-6-8)
    a. Drug absorption is delayed resulting in a slower onset of action occurring.
    b. There will be a decrease in body fluids, which will affect both drug concentrations and pharmacological effects.
    c. Enzyme concentrations within the liver will increase resulting in an increase in drug metabolism.
    d. The renal function decreases resulting in a slower drug elimination (excretion) rate.

20. Which of the following will *not* occur because of behavioral toxicity?(L-6-18)
    a. An individual may become less motivated.
    b. An individual will experience improved memory and learning functions.
    c. An individual's judgment may become distorted.
    d. An individual may experience a reduction in anxiety levels.

21. Which of the following drug classifications does not show a potential for possible drug dependence?(L-6-19)
    a. Amphetamines
    b. Antibiotics

    c. CNS stimulants
    d. Sedatives

22. Which of the following forms of drug dependence results in the development of physical symptoms when the drug is stopped?(L-6-19)
    a. Psychological dependence
    b. Physical dependence
    c. Tolerance
    d. All of the above

23. Which of the following is *not* an example of a parenteral route of administration?(L-6-14)
    a. Buccal
    b. Intrathecal
    c. Subcutaneous
    d. Topical

24. Which of the following terms refers to a drug that yields similar concentrations in the blood and tissues?(L-6-17)
    a. Biologically equivalent
    b. Chemically equivalent
    c. Therapeutically equivalent
    d. None of the above

25. Which of the following drug interactions occurs when one drug increases the potency or strength of another medication?(L-6-17)
    a. Additive effect
    b. Antagonism
    c. Potentiation
    d. Synergism

26. Which of the following terms refers to the process of converting a drug to a state, where it may be eliminated from the body?(L-6-6)
    a. Absorption
    b. Distribution
    c. Metabolism
    d. Elimination

27. Which of the following may occur as a birth defect if a pregnant woman takes lithium during pregnancy?(L-6-20)
    a. Cardiac defects
    b. CNS defects
    c. Feminization of the male fetus
    d. Masculinization of the female fetus

28. Which of the following is a synthetic reaction that occurs in the body during drug metabolism?(L-6-3, 6-6)
    a. Conjugation
    b. Hydrolysis

c. Oxidation

d. Reduction

29. Which of the following pregnancy categories reveal that teratogenic effects have been demonstrated in either women and/or animals?[L-6-20]

a. Pregnancy Category A

b. Pregnancy Category B

c. Pregnancy Category C

d. Pregnancy Category X

30. Which of the following terms will result in a decrease in the number of enzymes in the body during the metabolism of a drug?[L-6-3, 6-6]

a. Enzyme conjugation

b. Enzyme induction

c. Enzyme inhibition

d. Enzyme oxidation

True/False

Mark True or False for each statement. If it is false, correct the statement to make it true.

1. _____ The rate of absorption can be affected by its route of administration.[L-6-3, 6-4]

2. _____ It takes two half-lives for a drug to be eliminated from the body.[L-6-17]

3. _____ Nitroglycerin is administered sublingually because the route produces a higher concentration in the bloodstream than if it travels through the digestive tract.[L-6-14]

4. _____ It is extremely difficult to regulate a dose administered through inhalation methods.[L-6-14]

5. _____ A biologically equivalent drug produces similar concentrations in blood and tissues.[L-6-15, 6-17]

6. _____ A drug with a therapeutic equivalent code beginning with a "B" indicates that the drug is not therapeutically equivalent to other pharmaceutical products.[L-6-15]

7. _____ A medication that has been awarded a B code does not necessarily mean that the active ingredient is the cause of the problem but rather the dosage form.[L-6-15]

8. _____ The fetus is exposed to every drug that a woman takes during her pregnancy.[L-6-20]

9. _____ A patient described as hyperactive is one who experiences the desired effect at a low dosage.[L-6-10]

10. _____ Placebo drug effects are used during drug studies.[L-6-17]

11. _____ An idiosyncrasy is the usual effect associated with a drug.[L-6-10]

12. _____ An anaphylactic reaction may be fatal to an individual.[L-6-18]

13. _____ An additive effect is the combined effect of two drugs that has a combined effect greater than the sum of the two effects alone.[L-6-18]

14. _____ Some medications have the potential to be eliminated in the breast milk of a nursing mother.[L-6-20]

15. _____ Medications should always be taken on a full stomach to prevent stomach irritation.[L-6-14, 6-20]

Acronyms

Print the meaning of the following acronyms.[L-6-3, 6-16]

ADME _____

CDC _____

FDA _____

MTC _____

OTC _____

USAN _____

USP _____

Apply Your Knowledge

1. Using the *PDR* or *Drug Facts and Comparisons*, identify the different dosage forms for nitroglycerin, their strengths, and routes of administration. What conclusions can you make regarding dose and route of administration?[L-6-9, 6-14]

2. Using the *PDR* or *Drug Facts and Comparisons*, select an antibiotic and find the correct dosing for an infant, a child, an adult, a patient with liver problems, and a patient with kidney problems. What conclusions can you make regarding this medication?[L-6-9]

Antibiotic	Dosing
Infant	
Child	
Adult	
Patient with liver problems	
Patient with kidney problems	

3. A doctor prescribed the following medication for a patient:[L-6-8, 6-9]

   Zithromax #6
   Two caps stat, then one cap po d

   What type of dose is the first dose taken by the patient? _____

   Why would a physician prescribe it this way?
   _____

4. John Doe is prescribed Coreg 6.25 mg twice a day.[L-6-8]
   What would you call this type of dose?
   _____

5. Using the *PDR* or *Drug Facts and Comparisons*, make a list of foods that interact with Coumadin.[L-6-11]
   _____
   _____

6. A pharmacy patient is dropping off his prescription and you ask if he would like the generic medication if one were available. The patient asks what the difference is between the brand-name and generic medicines.[L-6-16]

   How do you respond? _____

7. What problem exists with prescribing Accutane to a pregnant woman?[L-6-20]
   _____

   Why? _____

8. A friend of yours consumes a minimum of 2 L of Mountain Dew daily. Today your friend consumes two 12-oz cans. Later in the day, she begins to experience severe headaches.[L-6-19] What is happening to your friend?
   _____

9. Identify the following terms in the Plasma concentration vs. Time graph shown below: onset of action, duration of action, termination of action, minimum effective concentration, and drug range.[L-6-9]

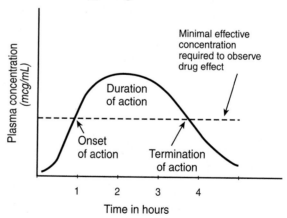

10. Using the *PDR* or *Drug Facts and Comparisons*, complete the following table.[L-6-9, 6-18]

Drug	Effect If Drug Concentration Is Below the Recommended Therapeutic Level	Effect If Drug Concentration Is Above the Recommended Therapeutic Level
Coumadin		
Dilantin		
Lithium carbonate		
Synthroid		

Practice Your Knowledge

Materials Needed

1. Legal pad
2. Pen or pencil

Goal

To become aware of the various warnings and drug interactions of OTC medications.[L-6-13, 6-18]

Assignment

1. Visit a local retail pharmacy and select a medication from each of the following categories.
2. Record the warnings found on the back of the box for each product.

Medication	Drug Interactions	Warnings
Advil		
Afrin Nasal Spray		
Aleve		
Alka-Seltzer		
Bayer Aspirin		
Benadryl		
Chlor-Trimeton		

Medication	Drug Interactions	Warnings
Claritin		
Cortaid		
Imodium AD		
Lotrimin		
Melatonin		
Metamucil		
Milk of Magnesia		
Mylanta		
Neosporin		
Pepcid AC		
Robitussin		
St. John's wort		
Sudafed		
Tavist-D		
Tylenol		
Vicks Cough Syrup		
Vitron C		
Zostrix		

Practice Your Knowledge

Materials Needed

1. Legal pad
2. Pen or pencil

Goal

To become aware of the active ingredients names, dosage forms, and routes of administration for various OTC medications.(L-6-14, 6-16)

Assignment

Visit a local pharmacy and identify the generic names, available dosage forms, and routes of administration for the following OTC medications.

Medication	Active Ingredient(s)	Available Dosage Form(s)	Route(s) of Administration
Advil			
Anusol			
Bayer Aspirin			
Benadryl			
Claritin			
Comtrex			
Cortaid			
Dimetapp			
Lotrimin			
Maalox			
Mylanta			
Neosporin			
Pepto Bismol			
Robitussin			
Tylenol			
Zyrtec			

Calculation Corner

A patient is prescribed cephalexin 500 mg every 6 hours.

How much medication remains after four half-lives? _____
(L-6-17)

Work Out the Solution

Pharm Facts—Research

Using either the *PDR* or *Drug Facts and Comparisons,* complete Table 6-1.

Table 6-1

Brand Name	Generic Name	List Five Adverse Effects	Nephrotoxicity (yes or no)	Hepatotoxicity (yes or no)	List Any Teratogenic Effects
Accutane					
Achromycin					
Bactrim					
Cipro					
Coumadin					
Diflucan					
Dilantin					
Epivir					
Eskalith					
Estrace					
Garamycin					
Lamisil					
Minocin					
Oxycontin					
Paxil					
Ritalin					
Sporanox					
Synthroid					
Vancocin					
Vasotec					
Vibramycin					
Wellbutrin					
Yaz					
Zestril					
Zithromax					

Did You Know?

The term *pharmacology* can be traced to the Greek term "pharmakon" meaning remedy or poison, as published in Plato's dialogues.[L-6-1]

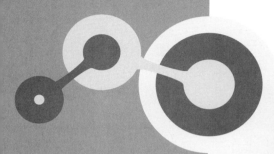

7

Drug Classifications

Learning Outcomes

Upon completion of this laboratory chapter, you will be able to:

L-7-1   Define the term *classification*.

L-7-2   List the reasons drug classifications are important to pharmacy technicians

L-7-3   Differentiate between agonists and antagonists.

L-7-4   Define and describe the role of neurotransmitters as they relate to drug action.

L-7-5   Classify medications or agents given a particular organ, system, or function.

L-7-6   Define *controlled substances*.

L-7-7   Identify drugs categorized as controlled substances.

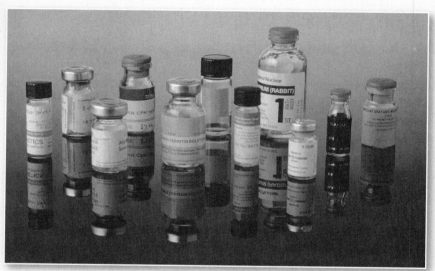

PTCB

In preparation for the certification examination, you should understand and perform activities associated with the following PTCB Knowledge Statement:

Domain I. Assisting the Pharmacist in Serving Patients

Knowledge of generic and brand names of pharmaceuticals (5)

Knowledge of therapeutic equivalence (6)

Knowledge of signs and symptoms of disease states (10)

Knowledge of drug indications (18)

Introduction to Drug Classifications^(L-7-1)

Medications are classified based upon therapeutic use and/or mechanism of action. Using knowledge of medication classification, the pharmacy technician is able to identify medications of the same therapeutic class or mechanism of action. This knowledge will also enable the technician to specify indications and potential contraindications for various pharmaceuticals. In summary, through knowledge of drug classifications, a technician may avert a medication error due to drug class duplication, recognize a potential drug–drug interaction, or identify a potential contraindication for the use of a particular drug (e.g., allergy).

Test Your Knowledge

Multiple Choice Questions

Answer the following multiple choice questions. When you have finished, check your answers and then review those areas that need improvement.

1. Which of the following medications is categorized by its mechanism of action?^(L-7-5)
   a. Minocycline
   b. Ibuprofen
   c. Cimetidine
   d. Penicillin

2. Which of the following medications is *not* an anticonvulsant medication?^(L-7-5)
   a. Diazepam
   b. Topiramate
   c. Carbamazepine
   d. Zolpidem

3. _____ is a situation in which a specific medication should not be administered.^(L-7-2)
   a. Indication
   b. Contraindication
   c. Drug interaction
   d. a and c

4. Which of the following medications is *not* an anti-Parkinson's medication?^(L-7-3, 7-4, 7-5)
   a. Tolcapone
   b. Levodopa
   c. Alprazolam
   d. Selegiline

5. Which of the following is an illicit drug of abuse?^(L-7-5, 7-6, 7-7)
   a. Penicillin
   b. Codeine
   c. Methamphetamine
   d. Ambien

6. Which of the following most likely given to a woman over the age of 55?^(L-7-5)
   a. Ortho-Tricyclen
   b. Prempro
   c. Ovcon-35
   d. Allese

7. Which of the following agents is used to treat gastrointestinal system disorders?^(L-7-5)
   a. Heparin
   b. Omeprazole
   c. Albuterol
   d. Adderal

8. Which of the following may be used to treat conditions affecting more than one system depending on dosage form?^(L-7-3, 7-5)
   a. Timolol
   b. Amiodarone
   c. Levothyroxine
   d. Glyburide

9. Which of the following medications is used to manage diabetes mellitus?(L-7-5)
   a. Nifedipine
   b. Propranolol
   c. Procainamide
   d. Pioglitazone

10. Which of the following is not an antipsychotic agent?(L-7-4, 7-5)
    a. Risperdone
    b. Haloperidol
    c. Albuterol
    d. Fluphenazine

11. Which of the following is an HMG-CoA reductase inhibitor?(L-7-5)
    a. Pravastatin
    b. Fluconazole
    c. Nystatin
    d. Methylprednisolone

12. Which of the following categories of medications is used in the management of HIV?(L-7-5)
    a. Protease inhibitors
    b. Catechol-O-methyltransferase inhibitors
    c. Angiotensin-converting enzyme inhibitors
    d. Nonsteroidal anti-inflammatory drugs

13. Which of the following medications is *not* a diuretic agent?(L-7-5)
    a. Furosemide
    b. Hydrochlorothiazide
    c. Amlodipine
    d. Triamterene

14. Which of the following agents is used to treat glaucoma?(L-7-3, 7-4, 7-5)
    a. Pilocarpine
    b. Ciprofloxacin
    c. Naphazoline
    d. Atropine

15. Which of the following categories of medications are antibiotics?(L-7-5)
    a. Histamine 2 receptor antagonists
    b. Beta blockers
    c. Macrolides
    d. Anticoagulants

16. The classification for drugs employed against human immunodeficiency virus (HIV) is called _____ (L-7-2, 7-4)
    a. antibiotics.
    b. antifungals.
    c. antiretrovirals.
    d. antihyperlipidemics.

17. Which of the following medications is *not* an antibiotic agent?(L-7-5)
    a. Azithromycin
    b. Ciprofloxacin
    c. Penicillamine
    d. Sulfamethoxazole

18. Which of the following agents is an ectoparasiticide?(L-7-5)
    a. Hydrocortisone
    b. Permethrin
    c. Benzoyl peroxide
    d. Naftifine

19. Which of the following is *not* an antiprotozoal medication?(L-7-5)
    a. Mefloquine
    b. Paromomycin
    c. Metronidazole
    d. Penicillin

20. Which of the following is *not* an ultra-rapid-acting insulin?(L-7-5)
    a. Insulin glulisine
    b. Insulin glargine
    c. Insulin aspart
    d. Insulin lispro

21. Which of the following is used in the management of helminthic infestations?(L-7-5)
    a. Mebendazole
    b. Fluconazole
    c. Ciclopirox
    d. Tolnaftate

22. A patient has presented to the pharmacy with a new prescription for Valium (diazepam). This drug is in the same category as_____ (L-7-2,7-5,7-6,7-7)
    a. phenobarbital.
    b. tolcapone.
    c. alprazolam.
    d. morphine.

23. A patient calls the pharmacy requesting refills on his Inderal (propranolol). While looking at the patient's medication profile, you notice he is also taking Ambien (zolpidem), Nitrostat sublingual (nitroglycerin), and Vasotec (enalapril). Which one of the medications from the profile is also used in the management of hypertension?(L-7-2, 7-5)
    a. Zolpidem
    b. Nitroglycerin
    c. Enalapril
    d. None of the above

24. Mary K comes into the pharmacy and mentions that she needs a refill on her osteoporosis medication, but forgot her bottle at home. As you check her profile you observe the following medications: flavoxate, candesartan, alendronate, and latanoprost. Which of the following is the agent for osteoporosis?[L-7-2, 7-5]
    a. Flavoxate
    b. Candesartan
    c. Alendronate
    d. Latanoprost

25. John D. presents a new prescription at the pharmacy window for isotretinoin. He mentions that he will want to talk to the pharmacist before starting to take the medication. What type of drug is isotretinoin?[L-7-2, 7-5]
    a. Antihypertensive
    b. Anti-acne
    c. Antihyperlipidemic
    d. Antihelmintic

Matching

Match the medication with its appropriate category.[L-7-5]

_____ 1. Inderal (propranolol)

_____ 2. Synthroid (levothyroxine)

_____ 3. Lipitor (atorvastatin)

_____ 4. Risperdal (risperdone)

_____ 5. Zoloft (sertraline)

_____ 6. Nexium (esomeprazole)

_____ 7. Levaquin (levofloxacin)

_____ 8. Allegra (fexofenadine)

_____ 9. Fosamax (alendronate)

_____10. Epogen (erythropoietin alfa)

A. Antibiotic

B. Antihyperlipidemic

C. Hematopoietic factor

D. Antihypertensive

E. Thyroid medication

F. Antipsychotic

G. Osteoporosis medication

H. Proton pump inhibitor

I. Antidepressant

J. Antihistamine

Apply Your Knowledge

1. For each drug provide the correct drug classification.[L-7-5]
    a. Amiodarone _____
    b. Nexium _____
    c. Celexa _____
    d. Aricept _____
    e. Lipitor _____
    f. Novolin _____
    g. Zyrtec _____
    h. Famvir _____
    i. Gleevec _____
    j. Actos _____

2. Go to Rx List—The Internet Drug Index, **www.rxlist.com**. Print the most recent Top 200 drug list. For each drug on the list, and from memory, classify each drug listed. How did you do?[L-7-2, 7-5]

3. As an additional exercise, work with a partner to classify each of the top 200 drugs and to identify brand name (if the generic is printed on the list) or generic name of each drug on the list. Check your work. In a few days, test each other on brand and generic and category of medication.[L-7-5]

Practice Your Knowledge

Materials Needed

1. Bottles of stock medications
2. Paper
3. Pencil
4. Timer or stopwatch

Goal

To demonstrate the ability to classify randomly selected medications, and to correctly replace the containers on the shelf.(L-7-1, 7-2, 7-5)

Assignment

1. Without watching, have a classmate randomly select 20 medication bottles from the shelves in the pharmacy laboratory. Your classmate then uses the timer or stopwatch to determine how long it takes you to classify or identify a particular disease state for which each agent is used. Another classmate can keep track of your responses on a sheet of paper.(L-7-5)
   Were you able to accurately classify each medication?
   How long did it take you to complete the task?
   Could you do better?
2. Now have the classmate reset the timer or stopwatch to determine how quickly you can place the bottles back on the shelf in the appropriate places.(L-7-2, 7-5)
   Are the bottles placed appropriately on the shelf?
   How long did it take you?
3. Switch places with your partner. Have him or her leave the room or turn around while you randomly pull 20 bottles from the shelf. Repeat the above exercises using the timer or stopwatch.(L-7-2, 7-5)

Evaluation Form

Practice the task until you are able to obtain a fair or excellent self-evaluation, then obtain a final evaluation from your instructor.

Task	Self-Evaluation			Instructor Evaluation		
	Rating			Rating		
	Excellent	Fair	Poor	Excellent	Fair	Poor
Variety of randomly selected agents						
Number of selected agents (20)						
Correct responses for identifying classifications of agents						
Timeliness of responses for identifying agents						
Pronunciation of agents and classifications						
Correct replacement of agents on the shelves						
Timeliness of replacement of agents						

Calculation Corner

You receive a prescription for Amoxil (amoxicillin) suspension 200 mg every 8 hours for 10 days. You have in stock Amoxil 125 mg/5 mL suspension and Amoxil 250 mg/5 mL suspension.

1. Which suspension will you use and why? _____ (L-7-2)

2. For the suspension you chose, calculate the milliliters required for each dose, total milliliters administered each day, and minimum quantity of suspension needed to prepare the prescription. _____

Work Out the Solution

Pharm Facts—Research

Choose a category of medications from the chapter in which you have interest; for example, antifungals or antihypertensives.

1. Provide brand and generic names of the agents currently available in this category and provide the indications for the use of these agents.(L-7-5)

2. Identify ways you might assist the pharmacist in providing quality pharmaceutical care to patients who are taking agents from this category.(L-7-1,7-2,7-5,7-7)

Did You Know?

According to the FDA, 7 in 10 prescriptions filled in the United States are for generic drugs. The FDA requires generic drugs to have the same quality and performance as the brand-name drugs.

When a generic drug product is approved, it has met rigorous standards established by the FDA with respect to identity, strength, quality, purity, and potency. Some variability can and does occur during manufacturing for both brand-name and generic drugs. When a drug, whether generic or brand name, is mass-produced, very small variations in purity, size, strength, and other parameters are permitted. The FDA puts limits on how much variability in composition or performance of a drug is acceptable.(L-7-2, 7-5)

8

Over-the-Counter (OTC) Agents

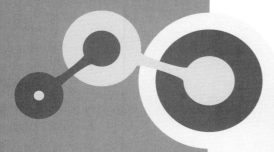

Learning Outcomes

Upon completion of this laboratory chapter, you will be able to:

L-8-1 Define *over-the-counter (OTC)* agents.

L-8-2 Identify the legal requirements for OTC agents.

L-8-3 Differentiate between OTC and prescription agents.

L-8-4 Differentiate between OTC drugs and dietary supplements.

L-8-5 Identify categories of OTC medications.

L-8-6 Classify OTC agents.

L-8-7 List common diagnostic agents/kits that are available OTC.

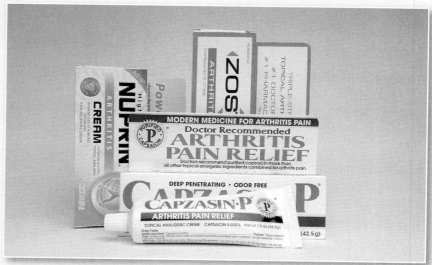

PTCB

In preparation for the certification examination, you should understand and perform activities associated with the following PTCB Knowledge Statement:

Domain I. Assisting the Pharmacist in Serving Patients

Knowledge of drug interactions (12)

Knowledge of effects of patient's age (14)

Knowledge of nonprescription (OTC) formulations (28)

Introduction to OTC(L-8-1, 8-2)

Over-the-counter (OTC) agents are available without prescription. There are other products, such as home diagnostic kits and dietary supplements, that are also available without a prescription. Because customers may ask questions about the various nonprescription agents, pharmacy technicians must be aware of the pharmacologic aspects of the agents, including indications, contraindications, and adverse drug reactions. Pharmacy technicians must also be aware of the packaging and proper storage of these agents to assist pharmacists and to communicate effectively with patients. The purpose of this laboratory chapter is to reinforce the students' understanding of nonprescription agents.

Test Your Knowledge

Multiple Choice Questions

Answer the following multiple choice questions. When you have finished, check your answers and then review those areas that need improvement.

1. Which of the following is *not* found on the label of OTC medications?(L-8-2)
   a. Appropriate dose
   b. Active ingredient(s)
   c. Storage instructions
   d. Alternative medications

2. Which of the following is a dietary supplement?(L-8-3)
   a. Vitamin C
   b. Aspirin
   c. Acetaminophen
   d. Ibuprofen

3. Agents that relieve pain are called(L-8-5)
   a. antipyretics.
   b. antipruritics.
   c. analgesics.
   d. anesthetics.

4. Agents that relieve fever are called(L-8-5)
   a. antiplatelets.
   b. analgesics.
   c. antipyretics.
   d. antiemetics.

5. Which of the following is an NSAID?(L-8-5)
   a. Acetaminophen
   b. Ibuprofen
   c. Aspirin
   d. Capsaicin

6. Which of the following categories of agents is employed against allergies?(L-8-5)
   a. Anesthetic
   b. Antiemetic
   c. Antihistamine
   d. Analgesic

7. Which of the following groups need not consult a physician or pharmacist prior to taking oral decongestants?(L-8-4, 8-5)
   a. Patients with diabetes
   b. Patients with hypertension
   c. Patients taking antidepressants
   d. Patients with bone disorders

8. Which of the following types of medications is not a gastrointestinal agent?(L-8-5)
   a. Laxatives
   b. Antiemetics
   c. Antifungals
   d. Antacids

9. Which of the following is an active ingredient in agents for sensitive teeth?(L-8-5)
   a. Fluoride
   b. Diphenhydramine
   c. Cimetidine
   d. Tetrahydrozoline

10. Which of the following types of ophthalmic preparations is *not* available over-the-counter?(L-8-2, 8-5)
    a. Anti-allergy
    b. Decongestant
    c. Artificial tears
    d. Antibiotic

11. An antitussive agent(L-8-5)
    a. relieves congestion.
    b. suppresses cough.
    c. decreases allergic reactions.
    d. decreases phlegm viscosity.

12. An antiemetic agent(L-8-5)
    a. increases defecation.
    b. decreases diarrhea.
    c. relieves hemorrhoidal discomfort.
    d. decreases nausea and vomiting.

13. Omeprazole is employed for relief in the _____ system.(L-8-5)
    a. respiratory
    b. gastrointestinal
    c. nervous
    d. genitourinary

14. Which of the following is *not* employed for fungal infections?(L-8-5)
    a. Clotrimazole
    b. Miconazole
    c. Hydrocortisone
    d. Tolnaftate

15. Which of the following is *not* an active ingredient in cough and cold preparations?(L-8-5)
    a. Pseudoephedrine
    b. Diphenydramine
    c. Dextromethorphan
    d. Methylcellulose

16. An excipient is the _____ in the dosage form.(L-8-4)
    a. active ingredient(s)
    b. inactive ingredient(s)
    c. label information
    d. packaging

17. Tamper-evident packaging includes all of the following *except*(L-8-1)
    a. glued box tops.
    b. shrink wrap.
    c. child safety caps.
    d. multiple layers of plastic wrap or packaging.

18. Which of the following is associated with Reye's syndrome?(L-8-5)
    a. Acetaminophen
    b. Aspirin
    c. Ibuprofen
    d. Pseudoephedrine

19. Which of the following is an active ingredient used in wart removal agents?(L-8-5)
    a. Salicylic acid
    b. Selenium sulfide
    c. Benzoyl peroxide
    d. Coal tar

20. Which of the following may be used for ear-wax removal?(L-8-5)
    a. Blistex
    b. Debrox
    c. Sominex
    d. Fostex

21. Which of the following is *not* an active ingredient in a nasal decongestant spray?(L-8-4, 8-5)
    a. Oxymetazoline
    b. Naphazoline
    c. Pseudoephedrine
    d. Phenylephrine

22. Which of the following is *not* a type of home diagnostic kit?(L-8-6)
    a. Pregnancy
    b. Ovulation
    c. Illicit drugs
    d. Dementia

23. Which of the following is *not* an antihistamine?(L-8-5)
    a. Claritin
    b. Tavist
    c. Prilosec OTC
    d. Benadryl

24. The active ingredient employed in smoking cessation products is _____(L-8-5)
    a. omeprazole.
    b. ibuprofen.
    c. benzocaine.
    d. nicotine.

25. Which of the following is *not* true regarding the administration of ophthalmic agents?(L-8-4, 8-5)
    a. Hands should be washed prior to administration.
    b. The tip of the dropper or applicator should not touch the eye.
    c. Patients should not see a physician if there is a foreign object in the eye.
    d. Patients who wear contact lenses should check with their eye health professional prior to using eye drops not designed for use with contact lenses.

Matching

Match the condition with the medication.[L-8-5]

_____ 1. Acne

_____ 2. Athlete's foot

_____ 3. Dandruff

_____ 4. Hemorrhoids

_____ 5. Alopecia

A. Selsun Blue

B. Fostex

C. Tinactin

D. Rogaine

E. Anusol

Match the active ingredient with its claim or use.[L-8-4, 8-5]

_____ 1. Guaifenesin

_____ 2. Pseudoephedrine

_____ 3. Dextromethorphan

_____ 4. Chlorpheniramine

_____ 5. Naphazoline

A. Oral decongestant

B. Nasal decongestant

C. Expectorant

D. Antitussive

E. Antihistamine

Apply Your Knowledge

1. In your own words, describe the process of a medication going from prescription to nonprescription. What federal agency is involved in this process?[L-8-2]

_____

_____

_____

_____

2. Name four nonprescription agents that were previously prescription only?[L-8-1, 8-2]

_____

_____

3. A patient approaches the counter and asks you, the pharmacy technician, what she should take for insomnia. How do you respond?[L-8-5]

_____

_____

4. You know Mrs. C. receives prescription medications for diabetes, as she has obtained these medications from your pharmacy for many years. She has a cold and has selected three cough and cold preparations she wishes to purchase. What do you do and why?[L-8-5]

_____

_____

5. Mr. B. has been receiving a prescription for Prilosec® (omeprazole) 20 mg for several years, and he picked up a refill yesterday. Today, he attempts to purchase Prilosec-OTC®. What do you tell Mr. B.?[L-8-5]

_____

_____

Practice Your Knowledge

Materials Needed

1. Large poster board
2. Markers
3. Empty packaging (boxes, bottles) of nonprescription agents
4. Glue
5. Tape

Goal

To be able to present an over-the-counter agent to the class and demonstrate knowledge and communication skills.(L-8-1, 8-2, 8-3, 8-6)

Assignment

1. Choose one over-the-counter medication for presenting to the class. There should be no duplication of agents among students.
2. Use empty over-the-counter boxes or containers to obtain information about the products.
3. Using the poster board and markers, write information about the medication including other brand names, generic name, indications, contraindications, precautions, adverse drug reactions, and dosing information. Also indicate why you chose this agent.
4. Glue the package or box onto the poster board.
5. Present the information to the class in 5 minutes and solicit questions following the presentation.(L-8-1)

Calculation Corner

Mrs. J. has run out of the Tylenol Children's Elixir (80 mg/2.5 mL) 1 teaspoonful four times daily as needed for fever for her son as directed by his pediatrician. After checking with the doctor, she comes in to the pharmacy for more Tylenol, but all you have available are the Tylenol Infant's Drops (80 mg/0.8 mL).

1. How many milliliters of Tylenol Infant's Drops should be given to Mrs. J.'s son in each dose? _____ (L-8-5)

Work Out the Solution

Pharm Facts—Research

Aspirin is often referred to as a wonder drug. Research the various uses for aspirin and the dosages necessary for each. Also find references indicating the drug interactions associated with aspirin.

1. Which prescription medications should not be taken with aspirin and why?(L-8-5)

_____

_____

_____

2. Which over-the-counter herbal preparations should not be taken with aspirin? (L-8-3)

_____

_____

_____

3. Find at least five over-the-counter products that contain aspirin and list them. (L-8-5)

_____

_____

_____

Did You Know?

The FDA offers an online resource, Medicines In My Home, a program that teaches consumers how to choose over-the-counter medicines and use them safely. (L-8-1)

The National Library of Medicine and the National Institutes of Health have an Internet site called Mediline Plus. Search for Over-the-Counter Medicine and review informational items provided such as a _Be MedWise_ quiz, a _Taking Medicines_ tutorial, and a _Over-the-Counter Sleep Medications_ video.

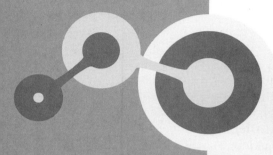

9

Complementary and Alternative Modalities

Learning Outcomes

Upon completion of this laboratory chapter, you will be able to:

L-9-1   Define *complementary* and *alternative medicine*.

L-9-2   Define *integrative medicine*.

L-9-3   List and describe types of complementary and alternative medicine.

L-9-4   List herbs employed in complementary and alternative medicine.

L-9-5   List other agents employed in complementary and alternative medicine.

L-9-6   List labeling requirements for dietary supplements.

L-9-7   Describe the role of the Food and Drug Administration in the safety of dietary supplements.

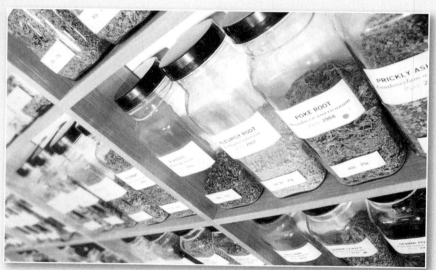

PTCB

In preparation for the certification examination, you should understand and perform activities associated with the following PTCB Knowledge Statement:

Domain I. Assisting the Pharmacist in Serving Patients

Knowledge of relative role of drug and nondrug therapy (e.g., herbal remedies, lifestyle modification, smoking cessation) (19)

Introduction to Complementary and Alternative Modalities(L-9-1)

Complementary and alternative modalities encompass all treatment modalities and/or practices of medicine except for Western or traditional medicine. Because integrative medicine involves the use of both traditional and complementary and alternative medicine, pharmacy technicians should be knowledgeable about both systems. As the use of complementary and alternative medicine increases in the United States, pharmacy staff members must commit themselves to keeping abreast of various treatments and herbal preparations that are carried in the pharmacy. In addition, because the pharmacy technician is often the first person a customer encounters when entering a pharmacy, he or she must be cognizant of the potential risks and benefits of the use of these products to properly refer patients to the pharmacist. This laboratory chapter is designed to enhance the pharmacy technician student's understanding of complementary and alternative treatments as they pertain to the practice of pharmacy.

Test Your Knowledge

Multiple Choice Questions

Answer the following multiple choice questions. When you have finished, check your answers and then review those areas that need improvement.

1. The consistency of components of the active ingredient from batch to batch and from manufacturer to manufacturer is called(L-9-7)
   a. adulteration.
   b. misbranding.
   c. standardization.
   d. contamination.

2. Which method of complementary and alternative medicine is based upon the principle that "like cures like"?(L-9-3)
   a. Ayurvedic medicine
   b. Chinese medicine
   c. Reiki
   d. Homeopathy

3. Which method involves the inhalation of certain oils to produce a desired effect?(L-9-3)
   a. Iridology
   b. Aromatherapy
   c. Rolfing
   d. Shiatsu

4. Which legislation defines dietary supplements and outlines their regulation?(L-9-7)
   a. DSHEA
   b. OBRA
   c. HIPAA
   d. DEA

5. The presence of impurities, microorganisms, pesticides, or radioactive substances in a product is referred to as(L-9-7)
   a. misbranding.
   b. contamination.
   c. standardization.
   d. none of the above.

6. In which method are adjustments of the spine made to relieve pressure and/or pain?(L-9-3)
   a. Iridology
   b. Aromatherapy
   c. Chiropractic medicine
   d. Homeopathy

7. Ayurvedic medicine is a(n)(L-9-3)
   a. ancient form of medicine originating in China involving herbal and animal source preparations to treat maladies.
   b. form of therapy that employs the use of cathartics and enemas to cleanse the colon.
   c. use of needles inserted into various areas (channels) of the body to restore balance.
   d. form of medicine originating in India that uses herbal preparations, dietary changes, exercises, and meditation to restore health and promote well-being.

8. Which of the following is *not* a form of alternative therapy?(L-9-1)
   a. Swedish massage
   b. Reiki
   c. Homeopathic preparations
   d. Western medicine

9. All herbal agents marketed in the United States are considered _____ (L-9-7)
   a. controlled substances.
   b. dietary supplements.
   c. over-the-counter drugs.
   d. prescription drugs.

10. Which of the following alternative modalities is used as a diagnostic tool?(L-9-1, 9-3)
    a. Chiropractic medicine
    b. Iridology
    c. Colonic therapy
    d. Chinese medicine

11. Which of the following is *not* a labeling requirement for dietary supplements?(L-9-6)
    a. Product must be identified as a dietary supplement, with the word "supplement"
    b. Statement of identity of product
    c. Supplement facts panel (including serving size, amount, and active ingredient)
    d. Date of manufacture

12. An increased risk of bleeding is a potential drug interaction resulting from the combination of _____ (L-9-2, 9-4)
    a. ginseng and decongestants.
    b. St. John's wort and anticoagulants.
    c. kava and sedatives.
    d. gingko and antiplatelet agents.

13. Increasing nervousness is a potential drug interaction that may result as a combination of _____ (L-9-2, 9-4)
    a. ginseng and decongestants.
    b. St. John's wort and sedatives.
    c. kava and antiplatelets.
    d. gingko and anticoagulants.

14. The combination of valerian with benzodiazepines may result in _____ (L-9-2, 9-4)
    a. increased nervousness.
    b. increased risk of bleeding.
    c. increased sedation.
    d. increased blood pressure.

15. A negative, nontherapeutic effect resulting from use of a medication is called _____ (L-9-1)
    a. drug interaction.
    b. contraindication.
    c. adverse drug reaction.
    d. none of the above.

16. Which of the following is *not* true regarding the use of herbal preparations?(L-9-4, 9-6, 9-7)
    a. Herbal preparations should not be used in pregnant or nursing women without consulting with a physician.
    b. Herbal preparations are safe because they are natural and nonsynthetic.
    c. Herbal preparations should not be used for life-threatening conditions.
    d. Herbal preparations should not be used in older people or small children without consulting a physician.

17. Which of the following herbs is considered unsafe for human ingestion, in any amount?(L-9-4, 9-7)
    a. Aloe
    b. Black cohosh
    c. Comfrey
    d. Dandelion

18. Which of the following does *not* exhibit sedative properties?(L-9-4)
    a. Kava
    b. Passionflower
    c. Valerian
    d. Senna

19. Which of the following should *not* be used in humans?(L-4, 9-7)
    a. Ginseng
    b. Wild yam
    c. Saw palmetto
    d. Snakeroot

20. Which of the following is *not* a fat-soluble vitamin?[(L-9-5)]
    a. Vitamin A
    b. Vitamin C
    c. Vitamin D
    d. Vitamin K

21. Which of the following is *not* a mineral?[(L-9-5)]
    a. Calcium
    b. Magnesium
    c. Arginine
    d. Phosphorus

22. Which of the following vitamins is administered for the prevention of neural tube defects?[(L-9-5, 9-6)]
    a. Vitamin A
    b. Niacin
    c. Vitamin C
    d. Folic acid

23. The primary claim of omega-3 fatty acids is that they _____[(L-9-5, 9-6)]
    a. reduce jet lag.
    b. relieve pain of osteoarthritis.
    c. slow the process of aging.
    d. reduce triglycerides.

24. An agent that is purported to have "probiotic" properties is _____[(L-9-5, 9-6)]
    a. glucosamine.
    b. DHEA.
    c. shark cartilage.
    d. lactobacillus.

25. Which of the following is thought to help manage symptoms of menopause?[(L-9-5, 9-6)]
    a. Chondroitin sulfate
    b. Melatonin
    c. Soy
    d. Ubiquinone

Matching

Match the agent with its claim or use.[(L-9-4)]

_____ 1. Black cohosh

_____ 2. Saw palmetto

_____ 3. Gingko

_____ 4. Aloe

_____ 5. St. John's wort

_____ 6. Valerian

_____ 7. Dandelion

_____ 8. Senna

_____ 9. Milk thistle

_____ 10. Guarana

A. Relief of prostate problems

B. Sedative

C. Mood stabilizer

D. Laxative

E. Increases energy

F. Enhances circulation

G. Liver protectant

H. Aids in wound healing

I. Increases urine output

J. Manages symptoms of menopause

Apply Your Knowledge

1. A patient has trouble falling asleep at night. Which herbal preparation(s) might be helpful for the patient?[(L-9-4, 9-6)]

    _____

2. Describe integrative medicine.[(L-9-2)]

    _____

    _____

3. Describe the difference between an over-the-counter medicine and a dietary supplement.(L-9-1)

_____

_____

4. Name a form of therapy that employs the use of enemas and cathartics to cleanse the colon and promote health.(L-9-3) _____

_____

_____

5. Describe chiropractic therapy.(L-9-3)

_____

_____

_____

6. _____ is defined as the consistency of components of the active ingredient from batch to batch and from manufacturer to manufacturer.(L-9-7)

7. What serious adverse effect may occur in a patient who is taking the anticoagulant Coumadin (warfarin) while taking gingko?(L-9-2, 9-4)

_____

_____

8. Name the agent that is a "probiotic" agent.(L-9-5)

_____

_____

9. Which dietary supplement may help relieve the pain associated with osteoarthritis?(L-9-5, 9-6)

_____

_____

10. _____ is a nonherbal dietary supplement that purports to reduce jet lag and insomnia.(L-9-5, 9-6)

Practice Your Knowledge

Material Needed

1. Bottles of dietary supplements for weight loss
2. Internet connection
3. Pens
4. Paper

Goal

Be able to review and analyze label information on products containing herbal agents for compliance with FDA regulations and consumer safety.(L-9-1, 9-7)

Assignment

1. Using at least three commonly marketed products for weight loss, examine the labeling information on the bottles for the proprietary blends. Write down the agents contained in the proprietary blends of at least three of the products. Do you see any similarities?(L-9-1, 9-4, 9-5, 9-6)

_____

_____

2. What differences do you see?(L-9-6)

_____

_____

3. Using the Internet, log on to the Web sites of these products. Do you think the claims are consistent with the labeling information?(L-9-6)

_____

_____

4. Do you think the claims are misleading in any way? Why? (L-9-6, 9-7)

_____

_____

5. Which groups of patients should avoid these products and why?(L-9-7)

_____

_____

Calculation Corner

Mr. Kline is a regular customer who today wishes to purchase a product containing 2 grain (gr) of rose hips.

1. How much is this in milligrams?

_____

Work Out the Solution

Pharm Facts—Research

Complete Table 9-1, using a Complementary and Alternative drug reference or the Internet. A good Internet site is the National Center for Complementary and Alternative Medicine (NCCAM). [L-9-4, 9-5, 9-6]

Table 9-1

Agent	Claim
	Appetite suppressant
Milk thistle	
	Increases circulation, improves memory
Coenzyme Q10	
	Enhances physical performance, builds lean body mass

Did You Know?

The flowering tops of St. John's wort are incorporated into capsules and teas.

Black snakeroot, bugbane, bugwort, and rattleweed are common names for black cohosh. [L-9-4]

Medication Management and Preparation

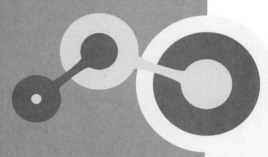

10

Dosage Forms and Routes of Administration

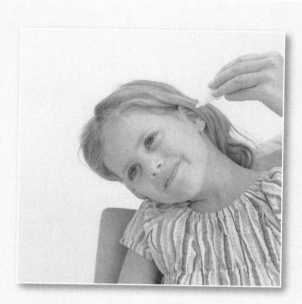

Learning Outcomes

Upon completion of this laboratory chapter, you will be able to:

L-10-1 Differentiate between the various routes of administration used in the practice of pharmacy.

L-10-2 Compare and contrast the various dosage forms used in pharmacy practice.

L-10-3 Explain the advantages and disadvantages of a particular dosage form.

L-10-4 Explain why a particular dosage form of a specific medication would be preferred over a different dosage form of the same medication.

L-10-5 Identify examples of each dosage forms.

L-10-6 Identify abbreviations associated with the various routes of administration and dosage forms.

PTCB

In preparation for the certification examination, you should understand and perform activities associated with the following PTCB Knowledge Statements:

Domain I. Assisting the Pharmacist in Serving Patients

Knowledge of pharmaceutical and medical abbreviations and terminology (4)

Knowledge of special directions and precautions for patient/patient's representative regarding preparation and use of medications (39)

Domain II. Maintaining Medication and Inventory Control Systems

Knowledge of dosage forms (4)

Introduction to Dosage Forms and Routes of Administration(L-10-6)

Every day in the practice of pharmacy a pharmacy technician processes prescriptions and/or medication orders. Often physicians use abbreviations in writing these orders and the pharmacy technician must know the meaning of them to fill the prescription properly. Many medications may be administered through different routes of administration and the pharmacy technician must understand the advantages and disadvantages of these routes of administration. In addition, some medications are available in multiple dosage forms and the technician must possess an understanding of these forms. It is extremely important that a pharmacy technician have a sound knowledge of pharmacy abbreviations, dosage forms, and their route of administration.

Test Your Knowledge

Multiple Choice Questions

Answer the following multiple choice questions. When you have finished, check your answers and then review those areas that need improvement.

1. Which of the following is *not* an advantage of an oral dosage form?(L-10-3)
   a. Easy to administer
   b. Inexpensive compared to other dosage forms
   c. Route is used for systemic effects
   d. Slower rate of therapeutic response

2. Which of the following is an advantage of the intravenous route of administration (may select more than one)?(L-10-3)
   a. Medications may not be either inactivated or destroyed in the GI tract
   b. Rapid absorption rate
   c. Quicker therapeutic response
   d. All of the above

3. Which of the following parenteral medications may use large volumes of medication to be infused?(L-10-1)
   a. Intradermal
   b. Intramuscular
   c. Intravenous
   d. Subcutaneous

4. Which of the following dosage forms may be administered topically?(L-10-4)
   a. Creams
   b. Lotions
   c. Ointments
   d. All of the above

5. Which of the following is an advantage of a patient taking a tablet (may select more than one)?(L-10-3)
   a. Accurate dosage of medication
   b. Dosage easily identifiable
   c. Ease of administration
   d. All of the above

6. Which of the following may be contained in a tablet?(L-10-3)
   a. Binders
   b. Diluents
   c. Disintegrants
   d. All of the above

7. Which of the following is an advantage of taking "extended-release medications"?(L-10-3)
   a. Good margin of safety
   b. Medication is used to treat chronic conditions
   c. Regular absorption from GI tract
   d. All of the above

8. Which of the following is an advantage of a capsule (may select more than one)?[L-10-3]
   a. Easily administered
   b. May contain multiple active ingredients
   c. Tasteless
   d. All of the above

9. Which of the following is *not* an advantage of transdermal drug delivery systems?[L-10-3]
   a. Avoidance of first-pass effect
   b. Avoidance of GI problems
   c. Therapy can be terminated quickly
   d. Used for potent drugs

10. Which of the following is a site of insertion for a suppository?[L-10-3]
    a. Rectum
    b. Urethra
    c. Vagina
    d. All of the above

11. Which of the following is *not* an advantage of a suppository?[L-10-3]
    a. Does not provide GI irritation
    b. Drug destruction due to acidic content of stomach is avoided
    c. Melts at body temperature
    d. Only select products are available for this route of administration

12. Which of the following may be dissolved in a solution?[L-10-3]
    a. Gas
    b. Liquid
    c. Solid
    d. All of the above

13. Which of the following dosage forms may contain an antiseptic, antibiotic, or anesthetic?[L-10-2, L10-3]
    a. Gargle
    b. Syrup
    c. Suspension
    d. All of the above

14. Which of the following is *not* a classification of an ingredient used in the preparation of a mouthwash?[L-10-2, L-10-3]
    a. Alcohol
    b. Flavoring
    c. Protectant
    d. Surfactant

15. Which of the following is *not* a method to prepare a medicated syrup?[L-10-2,10-3]
    a. Addition of sucrose to a prepared medicated liquid or a flavored liquid
    b. Condensation of a sucrose solution through evaporation
    c. Solution of the ingredients with the aid of heat
    d. Solution of the ingredients by agitation without the use of heat

16. Which of the following is *not* an advantage of an elixir?[L-10-3]
    a. Dosage can be adjusted to meet the needs of a patient
    b. Ease of administration
    c. May be either medicated or nonmedicated
    d. May not require the use of preservative in low concentrations (less than 10%)

17. How should a tincture be stored?[L-10-3]
    a. In a light-resistant container
    b. In a tightly closed container
    c. Away from high temperatures
    d. All of the above

18. Which of the following is *not* a disperse system?[L-10-2]
    a. Aerosol
    b. Emulsion
    c. Solution
    d. Suspension

19. Which of the following will determine whether an emulsion is oil-in-water or water-in-oil?[L-10-2, l-10-3]
    a. Desired effect
    b. Physical condition of the skin
    c. Therapeutic agent being used
    d. All of the above

20. Which is a characteristic of an emulsifying agent (may select more than one)?[L-10-2]
    a. Colorless
    b. Odorless
    c. Tasteless
    d. All of the above

21. Which of the following may affect an emulsion?[L-10-2, L-10-3]
    a. Air
    b. Bacteria
    c. Light
    d. All of the above

22. Which of the following is *not* a type of suspension?(L-10-2)
    a. Emulsion
    b. Lotion
    c. Magma
    d. Milk

23. Which of the following dosage forms must meet purity standards established by the USP?(L-10-2)
    a. Oral solutions
    b. Parenteral solutions
    c. Topical solutions
    d. Suppositories

24. Which of the following dosage forms cannot contain coloring agents?(L-10-3)
    a. Parenteral solutions
    b. Suspensions
    c. Syrups
    d. Topical solutions

25. Which parenteral dosage form may be referred to as a "ready-to-use" system?(L-10-2, 10-3)
    a. Large-volume parenteral
    b. Multiple-dose vial
    c. Single-dose vial
    d. Small-volume parenteral

26. Which of the following is an advantage for using an aerosol (may select more than one)?(L-10-3)
    a. Lower dosages
    b. Rapid onset of action
    c. Tamperproof
    d. All of the above

27. Which factor affects the use of an ophthalmic agent (may select more than one)?(L-10-3)
    a. Buffers
    b. Drug toxicity
    c. Isotonicity
    d. All of the above

28. Which of the following may occur if a pharmacy technician misinterprets a pharmacy abbreviation?(L-10-6)
    a. Adverse effects
    b. Poor patient compliance
    c. Prescription errors
    d. All of the above

29. Where does an enteric dosage form disintegrate?(L-10-3)
    a. In the intestine
    b. On the skin
    c. In the stomach
    d. Under the tongue

30. Where is a sublingual tablet administered?(L-10-2)
    a. In the lungs
    b. On the skin surface
    c. Beneath the skin
    d. Under the tongue

True/False

Mark True or False for each statement. If it is false, correct the statement to make it true.

1. _____ A sublingual dosage form is placed in the mouth between the cheeks.(L-10-2, 10-3)

2. _____ Oral medications cannot be used for patients in a coma.(L-10-1)

3. _____ Nitroglycerin is an example of a buccal medication used in the treatment of angina.(L-10-3)

4. _____ Rectal medications may be used for both local and systemic effects.(L-10-3)

5. _____ Parenteral injectable medications require the use of a syringe and a needle.(L-10-1)

6. _____ Parenteral injectable medications require a sterile compounding environment.(L-10-1)

7. _____ All tablets can be chewed.(L-10-3)

8. _____ Oral dosage forms are safer to use than parenteral dosage forms.(L-10-3)

9. _____ A size 5 capsule weighs more than a size 000 capsule.(L-10-2)

10. _____ A diluent is another term meaning active ingredient.(L-10-2)

11. _____ A disadvantage of extended-release products is "dose dumping."(L-10-3)

12. _____ Extended-release products possess the same mechanism of drug delivery.(L-10-3)

13. _____ There are two types of capsules: hard- and soft-shelled.(L-10-2)

14. _____ Transdermal drug delivery systems are used to place a drug in systemic circulation.(L-10-1, 10-3)

15. _____ An emulsion may be either oil-in-water or water-in-oil.(L-10-2)

16. _____ Solutions should be stored in tight containers and away from excessive heat.(L-10-2)

17. _____ A solution consists of three distinct phases.(L-10-2, 10-3)

18. _____ A solution may be diluted.(L-10-3)

19. _____ Solutions should be stored in light-resistant containers because the substances may begin to break down.(L-10-2, 10-3)

20. _____ Otic solutions must be prepared under sterile conditions.(L-10-3)

21. _____ Topical solutions always contain alcohol.(L-10-2)

22. _____ Oral dosage forms do not require the patient to possess any special skills to administer them.(L-10-3)

23. _____ A douche may be used to cleanse the eye.(L-10-3)

24. _____ Not all syrups are medicated.(L-10-2, 10-3)

25. _____ A syrup contains alcohol.(L-10-3)

26. _____ A sublingual dosage form bypasses the digestive system.(L-10-1)

27. _____ Emulsions are a stable dosage form.(L-10-3)

28. _____ Flexibility may be a problem with small-volume parenterals because one is unable to change either the concentration or volume.(L-10-3)

29. _____ A suspension may be used externally or internally depending on the medication.(L-10-3)

30. _____ Ophthalmic agents may provide either topical or systemic effects.(L-10-3)

31. _____ A capsule may be delay-released.(L-10-3)

32. _____ Emulsions are a two-phase system.(L-10-3)

33. _____ A suspension may be available for immediate use or reconstituted.(L-10-3)

34. _____ Parenteral suspensions do not need to meet USP–NF criteria for purity.(L-10-3)

35. _____ An IV is a parenteral dosage form.(l-10-3)

Abbreviations

Print the meaning of the following pharmacy abbreviations.(L-10-6)

aa	_____	mcg	_____
ac	_____	mEq	_____
ad lib	_____	mg	_____
am	_____	mL	_____
bid	_____	non rep	_____
caps	_____	oint	_____
dtd	_____	pc	_____
elix	_____	pm	_____
emuls	_____	prn	_____
gtt(s)	_____	qid	_____
hr	_____	rep	_____
hs	_____	Rx	_____
kg	_____	Sig	_____
lb	_____	sl	_____

sol   _____

stat   _____

syr   _____

tabs   _____

tbsp   _____

tid   _____

tsp   _____

ung   _____

vag   _____

Apply Your Knowledge

1. A patient has brought in a prescription requiring you to compound an ointment. The physician did not provide you with the name of an ointment base to use. How would you select the proper ointment base?(L-10-2, 10-3)

2. Both ointments and creams are topical preparations. Which do you prefer and why?(L-10-3)

3. A patient brings in a prescription to be compounded. You are instructed to add an equal volume of distilled water to a pint of stock solution. What would be the strength of the final product?(L-10-3)

4. If you were a parent of young child, would you administer an elixir to him or her? Why or why not?(L-10-3)

5. A patient receives a prescription for amoxicillin suspension. What auxiliary labels would you apply to the bottle and why?(L-10-3)

6. You have developed a headache while at work in the pharmacy. During your break, you purchase a bottle of Tylenol, which is available in a variety of dosage forms. Which dosage form of Tylenol would you select and why?(L-10-3)

7. A patient brings in a prescription for Phenergan 25 mg to treat nausea. Phenergan is available as a tablet, an elixir, an injection, and a suppository. Which of these dosage forms should the physician prescribe for the patient and why?(L-10-1, 10-3)

8. Amoxicillin 250 mg is available as an oral suspension, a chewable tablet, and a capsule. Which of the three dosage forms will result in the patient receiving therapeutic effect first? Why?(L-10-3)

9. What are the advantages of using an intravenous medication?(L-10-3)

10. Why do you think that the majority of medications are available as an oral dosage form?(L-10-3)

Practice Your Knowledge

Materials Needed

1. Paper
2. Pencil

Goal

To become familiar with the active ingredients contained in OTC medications, their dosage forms and routes of administration.

Assignment

Visit your local pharmacy and collect the following information on these over-the-counter (OTC) medications. (L-10-1, 10-2, 10-5)

OTC Medication	Active Ingredient(s)	Dosage Form(s)	Route of Administration
Afrin			
Aleve			
Benadryl			
Caladryl			
Claritin			
Contac			
Cortaid			
Debrox			
Delsym			
Epsom Salts			
Hold			
Imodium A-D			
Lamisil AF			
Medi-Plast			
Metamucil			
Monistat 7			
Mylanta			
Naphcon A			
Ocean			
Pepcid AC			
Pepto Bismol			
Preparation H			
Robitussin			
Tylenol			
Vitamin A			
Vitamin E			
Zantac			

Practice Your Knowledge

Material Needed

1. *Drug Facts and Comparisons* or *PDR*
2. Pen or pencil

Goal

To determine if the selected prescriptions can be dispensed as written.

Assignment

Review the following prescriptions. Can they be dispensed as written? If they cannot, indicate the error and correct it using the chart provided. (L-10-1, 10-5, 10-6)

Rx 1: Bactrim Elix   120 mL
       1 tsp po bid

Rx 2: Rowasa tab   #14
       1 tab po bid

Rx 3: Cortisporin Otic gtt 1 box
       1 gtt in left eye bid

Rx 4: Lipitor 10 mg tab   #30
       1 tab sl

Rx 5: Coumadin 5 mg   one month's supply
       Inject 5 mg IV q am

Rx 6: Heparin 10,000   one month's supply
       International Units
       1 tab po q am

Rx 7: Amoxicillin Elixir   250 mg/5 mL
       1 tsp po tid

Rx 8: Allegra D cap   #30
       1 cap po qd

Rx 9: Xalatan Syrup   1 bottle
       1 gtt in the affected
       eye qd

Rx 10: Humulin N Insulin   10 mL
       Suspension
       1 mL po qam

Prescription Number	Error	Correction
#1		
#2		
#3		
#4		
#5		
#6		
#7		
#8		
#9		
#10		

Calculation Corner

A patient presents you with the following prescription order:

Salicylic Acid   10%
Petrolatum qs   1 lb
Apply bid

1. How many grams of salicylic acid is required to prepare this compound?

(L-10-2)

Work Out the Solution

Pharm Facts—Research

Use *Drug Facts and Comparisons* or the *PDR* to complete Table 10-1. Indicate the route of administration for each dosage form available for each medication.[L-10-2, 10-3]

Table 10-1

Brand Name	Generic Name	Available Dosage Forms	Route of Administration for Each Dosage Form	Indication	List Five Side Effects
Advair					
Amoxil					
Biaxin					
Ciloxan					
Cipro					
Demerol					
Depakene					
Dilantin					
Dovenex					
Go-Lytely					
Haldol					
Lidex					
Minocin					
Mycostatin					
Proventil					
Reglan					
Rowasa					
Terazol					
Thorazine					
Zovirax					

Did You Know?

Many of the pharmacy abbreviations used today have their origin from Latin words.[L-10-6]

Extemporaneous and Sterile Compounding (IV Admixtures)

11

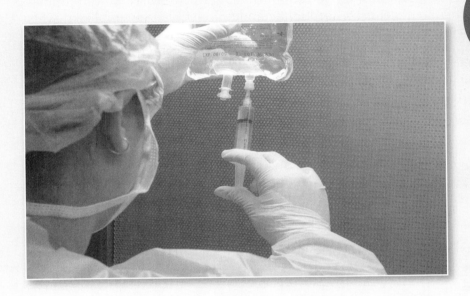

PTCB

In preparation for the certification examination, you should understand and perform activities associated with the following PTCB Knowledge Statement:

Domain I. Assisting the Pharmacist in Serving Patients

Knowledge of practice site policies and procedures regarding prescriptions or medication orders (20)

Knowledge of procedures to prepare IV admixtures (55)

Knowledge of procedures to prepare total parenteral nutrition (57)

Knowledge of procedures to prepare reconstituted injectable medications (58)

Knowledge of aseptic technique (65)

Knowledge of infection control procedures (66)

Learning Outcomes

Upon completion of this laboratory chapter, you will be able to:

L-11-1 Define *extemporaneous compounding*.

L-11-2 Define *sterile compounding*.

L-11-3 Identify types of products produced by sterile compounding.

L-11-4 Identify pharmacy settings where nonsterile compounding occurs.

L-11-5 Identify common pharmacy equipment or supplies used in extemporaneous compounding.

L-11-6 Articulate which types of preparations must be prepared using aseptic technique and which do not require aseptic technique.

L-11-7 Identify pharmacy settings where sterile compounding occurs.

L-11-8 Define *aseptic technique*.

(Continued)

Learning Outcomes *(Cont'd)*

L-11-9 Describe how aseptic technique relates to infection control.

L-11-10 Explain and describe the cleaning and use of the laminar flow hood.

L-11-11 Describe the use of personal protective equipment in sterile compounding.

L-11-12 Identify the regulations associated with sterile compounding.

Introduction to Extemporaneous and Sterile Compounding(L-11-1, 11-2)

Sterile compounding is the manufacture of pharmaceutical products requiring the use of aseptic technique; for example, the preparation of intravenous medications. Nonsterile (extemporaneous) compounding does not require aseptic technique; for example, the preparation of creams or ointments. Proper aseptic technique allows for the maintenance of product sterility. As sterile compounds are free of pathogens and contaminants, special care must be taken to preserve the sterility of these compounds for administration to patients. Products requiring sterile compounding include preparations to be administered intravenously, intramuscularly, and subcutaneously. Aseptic technique must also be employed when preparing medications that will be administered in the eye. Products for topical administration do not require aseptic technique. This laboratory chapter serves as a review of the major aspects of sterile and nonsterile compounding as they pertain to the responsibilities and duties of the pharmacy technician.

Test Your Knowledge

Multiple Choice Questions

Answer the following multiple choice questions. When you have finished, check your answers and then review those areas that need improvement.

1. Which of the following is *not* a route of administration requiring sterile compounding?(L-11-3)
   a. Intravenous
   b. Intramuscular
   c. Ophthalmic
   d. Topical

2. Another term for total parenteral nutrition is(L-11-3)
   a. reconstitution.
   b. hyperalimentation.
   c. enteral nutrition.
   d. none of the above.

3. Which of the following is a set of enforceable and official regulations governing sterile compounding?(L-11-9)
   a. USP<797>
   b. ASHP
   c. IVP
   d. IVPB

4. Pyrogens are defined as(L-11-6)
   a. fungi.
   b. fever-producing agents.
   c. bacteria.
   d. viruses.

5. For which of the following routes of administration is sterile compounding *not* required?(L-11-3)
   a. Intra-arterial
   b. Intravenous
   c. Oral
   d. Intrathecal

6. Sterile compounding may occur in all of the following pharmacy settings *except*(L-11-4)
   a. inpatient.
   b. home infusion.
   c. long-term care.
   d. all are potential sites for sterile compounding.

7. Which of the following is *not* one of the responsibilities of the pharmacy technicians in compounding?[(L-11-9)]
   a. Preparing and sorting labels
   b. Retrieving the materials needed for compounding
   c. Affixing the label to the packaging
   d. Writing the medication order

8. According to ASHP, the pharmacy is responsible for ensuring that sterile compounded products are[(L-11-3, 11-9)]
   a. free from contaminates.
   b. therapeutically appropriate.
   c. properly labeled.
   d. all of the above.

9. The laminar flow hood should be turned on for at least _____ before compounding begins.[(L-11-7)]
   a. 10 minutes
   b. 15 minutes
   c. 30 minutes
   d. 45 minutes

10. Which of the following is a type of non-disposable equipment used in sterile compounding?[(L-11-8)]
    a. Gloves
    b. IV additive machines
    c. Syringes
    d. Needles

11. The airflow in laminar flow hoods is either vertical or[(L-11-7)]
    a. horizontal.
    b. diagonal.
    c. circular.
    d. none of the above.

12. Which of the following is a disposable item used in nonsterile compounding?[(L-11-2)]
    a. Parchment paper
    b. Laminar flow hood
    c. Class A balance
    d. Automated pumps

13. Which of the following is *not* a form of personal protective equipment?[(L-11-8)]
    a. Gown
    b. Mask
    c. Needle
    d. Gloves

14. Reconstitution involves[(L-11-1, 11-2)]
    a. placing a light-resistant bag over the final compounded product.
    b. adding diluent to a powder for suspension or dissolution.
    c. using a mortar and pestle to reduce particle size.
    d. none of the above.

15. The pharmacy technician begins aseptic technique by[(L-11-6)]
    a. thorough and proper hand washing.
    b. watching others use the laminar flow hood.
    c. checking the temperature of the refrigerator.
    d. affixing labels to the final product.

16. The laminar flow hood must be[(L-11-6, 11-7)]
    a. turned off at the end of each shift.
    b. cleaned using 70% isopropyl alcohol.
    c. cleaned using sterile water.
    d. cleaned only once a day.

17. A _____ needle must be used when transferring liquid from an ampule to an IV bag.[(L-11-3)]
    a. vented
    b. regular
    c. filtered
    d. hypodermic

18. Trituration involves _____[(L-11-3)]
    a. diluting powders.
    b. grinding particles.
    c. incorporating particles.
    d. filtering particles.

19. Which of the following parts of the laminar flow hood should *not* be cleaned by the pharmacy technician?[(L-11-7)]
    a. The horizontal working surface
    b. The Plexiglas sides
    c. The HEPA filter
    d. None of the above

20. Sepsis refers to[(L-11-6)]
    a. proper hood cleaning.
    b. proper aseptic technique.
    c. an interaction causing precipitation.
    d. an infection in the bloodstream.

21. Which of the following is *not* a component of TPN?(L-11-3)
    a. Lipids
    b. Antibiotics
    c. Dextrose
    d. Amino acids

22. Sterile compounding of chemotherapeutic agents requires the use of(L-11-4, 11-7)
    a. a vertical laminar flow hood.
    b. proper aseptic technique.
    c. proper hazardous waste disposal.
    d. all of the above.

23. Gowns used while compounding sterile products should have(L-11-8)
    a. short sleeves.
    b. no sleeves.
    c. an open front.
    d. a closed front.

24. Torn or damaged personal protective equipment(L-11-8, 11-9)
    a. can be worn until the end of the shift.
    b. should be replaced after the technician completes compounding.
    c. should be changed immediately.
    d. none of the above.

25. The pharmacy technician should *not*(L-11-5, 11-6)
    a. speak or cough into the hood.
    b. work at least 6 inches in the hood.
    c. arrange vials to ensure proper airflow in the hood.
    d. wash hands although gloves will be worn.

True/False

Mark True or False for each statement. If it is false, correct the statement to make it true.

1. _____ The pharmacy technician should clean all equipment used for compounding immediately after use.(L-11-1, 11-2)

2. _____ It is not necessary for the pharmacy technician to document that he or she cleaned the hood.(L-11-6, 11-7)

3. _____ Hair covers should be worn to keep hair away from the sterile compounding area. (L-11-8)

4. _____ Needles should not be recapped or broken.(L-11-6)

5. _____ The sharps container may be used to dispose of all pharmacy trash or debris including plastic wrap and syringe caps.(L-11-4, 11-9)

6. _____ The pharmacy technician should compound at least four orders at a time to decrease time spent compounding.(L-11-3)

7. _____ Thorough cleaning of the laminar flow hood involves removing the back screen and cleaning the HEPA filter.(L-11-7)

8. _____ Personnel training and competence are areas addressed in USP <797>.(L-11-9)

9. _____ Gloves should always be worn while compounding.(L-11-8)

10. _____ IV solutions should be checked for particulate matter after labeling.(L-11-2, 11-3)

Apply Your Knowledge

1. _____ is an enforceable set of guidelines governing sterile compounding.(L-11-9)

2. _____ is the organization that accredits health care organizations.(L-11-9)

3. TPN preparations may include _____, in addition to lipids, dextrose, and amino acids.(L-11-3)

4. Gowns used while compounding should have a(n) _____ front.(L-11-8)

5. Ampules should be broken carefully to minimize _____.(L-11-5, 11-6)

Practice Your Knowledge

Materials Needed

1. Gloves
2. Gown
3. Hair cover
4. Isopropyl alcohol spray and/or wipes
5. Laminar flow hood
6. Large-volume IV fluid bag
7. Low-lint towels
8. Mask
9. Needles
10. Seals
11. Syringes (10 mL)
12. Vials of sterile water

Goal

To demonstrate proper aseptic technique when performing intravenous admixture.(L-11-2, 11-5, 11-6, 11-7)

Assignment

1. Wash hands thoroughly using the proper technique.(L-11-6)
2. Prepare for working in the hood by donning personal protective equipment.(L-11-8)
3. Clean the laminar flow hood including the work area and the Plexiglas sides.(L-11-7)
4. Retrieve necessary supplies including syringes, needles, large-volume bag, and vial of sterile water.(L-11-2, 11-3)
5. After placing items in the hood, clean surfaces with isopropyl alcohol.(L-11-6)
6. Prepare syringe and needle by placing the needle on the syringe inside the laminar flow hood.
7. Pull the plunger back to 5 mL.(L-11-6)
8. Place the needle (bevel side up and at a 45-degree angle) on the rubber stopper of the vial of sterile water.(L-11-6)
9. Raise the syringe to a 90-degree angle immediately prior to inserting the needle into the vial of sterile water.(L-11-6)
10. Slowly inject the 5 mL of air into the vial.(L-11-6)
11. Invert the vial, and withdraw 5 mL of sterile water in the syringe.(L-11-6)
12. Withdraw the syringe from the vial.(L-11-6)
13. Inject the 5 mL of water into the large-volume IV bag.(L-11-6)
14. Place a seal on the injection port of the IV bag.(L-11-6)
15. Properly dispose of needles and discard empty vials.(L-11-9)

Evaluation Form

Practice the task until you are able to obtain a fair or excellent self-evaluation, then obtain a final evaluation from your instructor.

Task	Self-Evaluation			Instructor Evaluation		
	Rating			Rating		
IV Admixtures	Excellent	Fair	Poor	Excellent	Fair	Poor
Hand washing technique						
Proper donning of personal protective equipment						
Checking that laminar flow hood has been on for at least 30 minutes prior to working in the hood						
Thoroughness of cleaning the laminar flow hood						
Selection of items for working in the hood						
Cleaning of vials, bags, and puncture points in the hood						
Correct replacement of agents in the hood						
Technique in withdrawing the sterile water from the vial						
Technique employed while injecting the sterile water into the IV bag						
Placement of seal on the IV bag						
Disposal of syringe and needle in a sharps container						
Disposal of empty vials						

Calculation Corner

1. You receive an order to prepare 20 capsules containing 120 mg each of ascorbic acid.

   What is the total amount (in grams) of ascorbic acid required to complete the order?_____ (L-11-3)

2. You receive an order to prepare an IV piggyback for Gentamicin 60 mg. The pharmacy stocks Gentamicin 40 mg/mL._____ (L-11-2, 11-3)

   How many milliliters of Gentamicin will you add to the IV bag?_____ (L-11-6)

Work Out the Solution

Pharm Facts—Research

Lasix (furosemide) is a loop diuretic that is frequently administered via oral and parenteral routes.

1. Using pharmacy references, find the indications for furosemide, and be prepared to discuss conditions warranting parenteral administration instead of oral administration. (L-11-3)

2. Also look up potential risks and adverse reactions that may occur from rapid diuresis with this agent. Present your findings in class for discussion. (L-11-3)

Did You Know?

The FDA knows of more than 200 adverse events involving 71 compounded products since 1990. Some of these instances had devastating repercussions.

- Three patients died of infections stemming from contaminated compounded solutions that are used to paralyze the heart during open-heart surgery. the FDA issued a warning letter in March 2006 to the firm that compounded the solutions. (L-11-6)
- Two patients at a Washington, DC, Veterans Affairs hospital were blinded, and several others had their eyesight damaged by a compounded product used in cataract surgery. The product was contaminated with bacteria. In August 2005, the FDA announced a nationwide recall of this Trypan Blue Ophthalmic Solution. Contaminated solution had been distributed to hospitals and clinics in eight states. (L-11-4, 11-6)
- In March 2005, the FDA issued a nationwide alert concerning a contaminated compounded magnesium sulfate solution that caused five cases of bacterial infections in a New Jersey hospital. A South Dakota patient treated with the product developed sepsis and died. (L-11-5, 11-6)

Source: **www.fda.gov/ForConsumers/ConsumerUpdates/ucm107836.htm#flags.**

Medication Errors

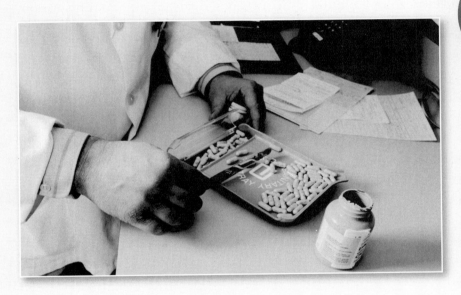

PTCB

In preparation for the certification examination, you should understand and perform activities associated with the following PTCB Knowledge Statements:

Domain I. Assisting the Pharmacist in Serving Patients

Knowledge of pharmaceutical, medical, and legal developments which impact on the practice of pharmacy (2)

Knowledge of techniques for detecting prescription errors (25)

Knowledge of quality improvement methods (49)

Domain III. Participating in the Administration and Management of Pharmacy

Knowledge of quality improvement standards and guidelines (10)

Learning Outcomes

Upon completion of this laboratory chapter, you will be able to:

L-12-1 Define *error* according to the institute of Medicine (IOM).

L-12-2 Identify types of medication errors.

L-12-3 Identify causes of medication errors.

L-12-4 Identify common prescribing errors observed by pharmacists.

L-12-5 Recognize costs associated with medication errors.

L-12-6 List methods to reduce medication errors.

L-12-7 Explain the NCC MERP index for categorizing medication errors.

L-12-8 Explain the problems identified by ISMP and solutions to these problems.

L-12-9 State the IOM's recommendations to improve patient safety.

L-12-10 Identify ways the patient can assist in reducing prescription errors.

(Continued)

Learning Outcomes *(cont'd)*

L-12-11 Differentiate between the types of dispensing errors.

L-12-12 Explain why there is not a valid defense for a prescription error.

L-12-13 Identify a "high-alert medication."

L-12-14 Explain National Patient Goals that have been established by The Joint Commission (TJC).

L-12-15 Discuss e-prescribing.

L-12-16 Identify the various agencies that oversee the reporting of medication errors and the processes that have been established to do so.

Introduction to Medication Errors(L-12-1)

The Institute of Medicine (IOM) defines an error as a "failure of a planned action to be completed as intended or the use of a wrong plan to achieve an aim." A medical error can occur in many different forms, such as diagnostic, technical, or even wound infection. Unfortunately, the largest cause of medical errors involves medication. According to the National Coordinating Council for Medication Error Reporting and Prevention, a medication error is "any preventable event that may cause or lead to inappropriate medication use or patient harm, while the medication is in the control of health care professional, health care product, procedures, and systems, including prescribing; order communication; product labeling, packaging, nomenclature; compounding; dispensing; distribution; administration; education; monitoring; and use." In other words, there are many different causes contributing to medication errors.

As a pharmacy technician, you will fill many prescriptions every day. Every time you fill a prescription, there is a possibility that an error may occur. It is extremely important to take the proper steps to reduce the number of possible prescription errors.

Test Your Knowledge

Multiple Choice Questions

Answer the following multiple choice questions. When you have finished, check your answers and then review those areas that need improvement.

1. Which of the following would be considered a prescription error?(L-12-2)
   a. Dispensing an incorrect medication to a patient
   b. Dispensing the incorrect strength of medication to a patient
   c. Identifying the incorrect route of administration of medication to the patient
   d. All of the above

2. Which category of error would occur if amoxicillin 500 mg is prescribed for a patient, but 250 mg of amoxicillin is dispensed instead. During patient counseling, the pharmacist notices the error and corrects it.(L-12-7)
   a. Category A
   b. Category B
   c. Category C
   d. Category D

3. A terminally ill patient is ordered 0.1 mL (2 mg) of morphine every 2 hours as needed. The patient receives two 1-mL doses. The patient dies. It cannot be determined if the patient died due to the morphine or due to the illness. What category of error is this?[(L-12-7)]
   a. Category G
   b. Category H
   c. Category I
   d. No error is committed

4. Who may commit a prescription error?[(L-12-3)]
   a. Nurse
   b. Pharmacist
   c. Physician
   d. Anybody

5. Which of the following is considered a prescribing problem?[(L-12-3)]
   a. Incorrect strength
   b. Patient allergy
   c. Route of administration is not indicated
   d. All of the above are considered prescribing problems

6. Which of the following pharmacy design factors can assist in reducing medication errors?[(L-12-6)]
   a. Ergonomic features
   b. Proper lighting
   c. Proper noise levels
   d. All of the above

7. What results would be observed by modifying prescription pads currently being used?[(L-12-6)]
   a. Cost containment of prescription pads
   b. Prescriptions would be uniform in size and would require less space for pharmacy storage
   c. Reduction of prescription problems and omissions errors
   d. All of the above

8. Which type of prescription error is the most common?[(L12-2, 12-4)]
   a. Improper dose
   b. Omission errors
   c. Prescribing errors
   d. Wrong route of administration

9. According to **MEDMARX**, which of the following contributes to most prescription errors?[(L-12-3)]
   a. Communication
   b. Computer entry
   c. Knowledge deficit
   d. Performance deficit

10. According to the *USP*, which of the following causes of medication errors is knowledge based?[(L-12-3)]
    a. Human
    b. Organizational
    c. Technical
    d. All of the above

11. Which of the following could result from a prescription error?[(L-12-5)]
    a. Death to the patient
    b. Physical injury to the patient
    c. Legal consequences for the person responsible for the error
    d. All of the above

12. Which of the following is a valid defense for committing a prescription error?[(L-12-12)]
    a. Excessive interruptions during the shift
    b. Lack of proper pharmacy staffing
    c. Inability to read the prescription
    d. None of the above

13. Which of the following are goals of TJC (formerly JCAHO) to improve patient safety in the hospital?[(L-12-14)]
    a. Eliminate wrong site, wrong patient, and wrong procedure surgery
    b. Improve the accuracy of patient identification
    c. Improve the effectiveness of communication among caregivers
    d. All of the above

14. Which of the following organizations conducts research on medication errors?[(L-12-16)]
    a. ISMP
    b. TJC, formerly JCAHO
    c. USP
    d. All of the above

15. Which organization has issued a "Do Not Use List" for pharmacy abbreviations and symbols?[(L-12-16)]
    a. ISMP
    b. TJC, formerly JCAHO
    c. USP
    d. All of the above

16. What practice is used the most upon discovery of a prescription error?[(L-12-8)]
    a. Informing the employee of the error
    b. Informing the patient of the error
    c. Initiating policy/procedure change
    d. Providing education training

17. What practice is used the least upon the discovery of a prescription error?(L-12-8)
    a. Informing the employee of the error
    b. Informing the patient of the error
    c. Initiating policy/procedure change
    d. Providing education training

18. Which of the following may cause prescription errors?(L-12-3, 12-4)
    a. Abbreviations and symbols used in prescriptions
    b. Medications, which may be spelled or sound similar to other medications
    c. Specific categories of medications
    d. All of the above

19. Which of the following categories may cause serious harm to a patient?(L-12-13)
    a. Chemotherapeutic agents
    b. Hypoglycemic agents
    c. Total parenteral solutions (TPNs)
    d. All of the above

20. Which of the following medications have a tendency to cause injury to a patient if used incorrectly?(L-12-13)
    a. Heparin
    b. Insulin
    c. Warfarin
    d. All of the above

21. What units should be used in writing out a prescription?(L-12-8)
    a. Apothecary
    b. Avoirdupois
    c. Metric
    d. All of the above

22. What should a pharmacy technician do if information on a prescription is missing?(L-12-4)
    a. Ask the patient if the physician provided him or her with the information
    b. Ask the pharmacist if he or she is familiar with the physician's prescribing habits
    c. Contact the physician for clarification
    d. All of the above

23. Which of the following is an advantage of electronic prescribing (may select more than one)?(L-12-15)
    a. Improvement of patient safety
    b. Patient convenience

    c. Reduction in the amount of time spent on prescription clarification
    d. All of the above

24. Which of the following practices may prevent medication dispensing errors?(L-12-6)
    a. Minimize distractions, such as interruptions
    b. Provide features to minimize fatigue, such as rubber mats on the floor to reduce stress on the legs
    c. Provide proper staffing during peak time periods
    d. All of the above

25. What is the minimum number of times a prescription label should be read before dispensing?(L-12-6)
    a. One time
    b. Two times
    c. Three times
    d. Four times

26. Which of the following is an advantage of e-prescribing?(L-12-15)
    a. Increased efficiency
    b. Increased patient safety
    c. Increased quality care
    d. All of the above

27. Which of the following pieces of information is required to be present when scanning bar codes?(L-12-6)
    a. Expiration date
    b. Lot number
    c. NDC number
    d. All of the above

28. Which of the following are steps in developing CQI for a pharmacy?(L-12-9)
    a. Reporting the details of the incident
    b. Understanding the incident
    c. Making recommendations for improvement
    d. All of the above

29. Which organization oversees MedWatch?(L-12-16)
    a. FDA
    b. ISMP
    c. TJC, formerly JCAHO
    d. All three organizations work together

30. What type of medications does VAERS monitor?(L-12-16)
    a. Injectable drugs
    b. Investigational drugs

c. Vaccines
d. All of the above

31. Who utilizes MEDMARX?(L-12-16)
    a. Chain pharmacies
    b. Franchise pharmacies
    c. Hospitals
    d. Independent pharmacies

32. What are the end results of organizations utilizing MEDMARX?(L-12-16)
    a. Elimination of costs associated with medication errors
    b. Improved patient safety
    c. Prevention of medication errors
    d. All of the above

33. What types of errors are reported to MERP?(L-12-16)
    a. Misadministration
    b. Miscalculations

c. Misinterpretations
d. All of the above

34. What can patients do to help reduce prescription errors?(L-12-10)
    a. Know their pharmacist
    b. Know the medications, both prescription and OTC, they are taking
    c. Use one pharmacy
    d. All of the above

35. Which of the following occur using the MEDMARX system?(L-12-16)
    a. Documentation
    b. Reporting analysis
    c. Tracking of medication errors
    d. All of the above

True/False

Mark True or False for each statement. If it is false, correct the statement to make it true.

1. _____ The abbreviations AD, AS, and AU have been mistaken for OD, OS, and OU.(L-12-8)

2. _____Only pharmacists are permitted to counsel patients.(L-12-6, 12-9)

3. _____ The use of bar codes does not significantly reduce prescription errors.(L-12-6, 12-8)

4. _____ A "safe rate" of filling prescriptions has been established for pharmacists and pharmacy technicians with one year of experience.(L-12-12)

5. _____ Punishment is an effective tool to prevent medication errors.(L-12-6)

6. _____ Using scannable bar codes can guarantee that the correct drug and dosage form are being administered to the correct patient.(L-12-6)

7. _____ If a prescription error occurs, the pharmacist will be found guilty of negligence because he or she did not act prudently in the processing of the prescription.(L-12-12)

8. _____ An institution is responsible for designing its pharmacy system. The system should improve the safety of the system and the outcomes associated with the system.(L-12-8)

9. _____ MedWatch and the MedWatch E-List provide the public with information regarding medication recalls and label changes.(L-12-16)

10. _____ MEDMARX allows for an individual to anonymously report adverse drug events.(L-12-16)

11. _____ It is illegal to e-prescribe Schedule II medications.(L-12-15)

12. _____ Proper staffing of the pharmacy may reduce prescription errors.(L-12-6)

Acronyms

Write the meaning of the following acronyms.(L-12-16)

APhA _____   MERP _____
CDC _____   NCVIA _____
CQI _____   PDCA _____
IOM _____   TQM _____
ISMP _____   VAERS _____

Apply Your Knowledge

Identify the error in each prescription.(L-12-4)

Rx 1:	Hydrochlorothiazide 50 mg 1 tab po at q hs Refill × 5	#30
Rx 2:	Ambien 10 mg (Note: Controlled substance) 1 tab po q hs prn insomnia Refill × 6	#30
Rx 3:	Nitroglycerin 1/150 gr 1 tab po qd prn angina Refill × 5	#25
Rx 4:	Lipitor 10 mg UD Refill × 5	#30
Rx 5:	Demerol 200 mg 1 tab po q 4 hours prn pain Refill	#20
Rx 6:	Anusol HC Supp 1 supp po q 4–6 hrs prn hemorrhoids Refill 1	#12
Rx 7:	Amoxicillin 250 mg/5 mL 1 tsp IV q 8 hrs Refill prn	150 mL
Rx 8:	Prednisone 5 mg 1 tab po qd for 5 days, then 1 tab po bid for 5 days, then 1 tab po tid for 5 days, then 1 tab po qid prn respiratory problems	#100
Rx 9:	Ibuprofen 800 mg 1 tab po q 4 hrs on an empty stomach Refill × 1	#30
Rx 10:	Cortisporin Otic Soln 1 gtt ou prn ear infection Refill	8 mL

Practice Your Knowledge

Material Needed

1. ISMP List of Confused Names (**www.ismp.org**)

Goal

To become familiar with medications that have been the source of medication errors due to the similarity in their names.(L-12-8)

Assignment

Using the ISMP List of Confused Names (**www.ismp.org**), identify all of the drugs that may be mistaken for the one given in the following table.(L-12-8, 12-13)

Medication Prescribed	Confused Drug Names
Amaryl	
Celebrex	
Celexa	
Clozaril	
Coumadin	
Cozaar	
Depakote	
Diovan	
Diprivan	
Estratest	
Humulin	
Inderal	
Kaletra	
Lanoxin	
Lasix	
Lexapro	
Lodine	
Maxzide	
Metformin	
Myleran	
Numega	
Pamelor	
Paxil	
Percocet	
Prilosec	
Protonix	
Reminyl	
Ritalin	
Roxanol	
Serafem	
Tegretol	
Tequin	
Tobradex	
Tylenol	
Wellbutrin	
Zebeta	
Zyprexa	
Zyrtec	
Zyvox	

Calculation Corner

1. A patient is to receive an IV infusion at a rate 100 mL/hr.
   How long would it take to infuse 1 liter of fluid?

   _____ (L-12-6)

   Work Out the Solution

Pharm Facts—Research

Use the *PDR* or *Drug Facts and Comparisons* to complete Table 12-1.(L-12-4, 12-6)

Table 12-1

Brand Name	Generic Name	Strengths	Indications	Contraindications	Adverse Effects
Ancobon					
Combivir					
Crixivan					
Diflucan					
Epivir					
Flumadine					
Fuzeon					
Hivid					
Invirase					
Lamisil					
Lexiva					
Loprox					
Nizoral					
Norvir					
Rescriptor					
Retrovir					
Sporanox					
Sustiva					
Symmetrel					
Terazol					
Trizivir					
Valtrex					
Videx					

Brand Name	Generic Name	Strengths	Indications	Contraindications	Adverse Effects
Viracept					
Viramune					
Viread					
Zerit					
Zovirax					

Did You Know?

A failure to follow hospital policies and procedures contributed to the accidental overdose of actor Dennis Quaid's twins at the hospital.

Heparin 10-unit vials and 10,000-unit vials were being stored in the same hospital drawer.[L-12-3]

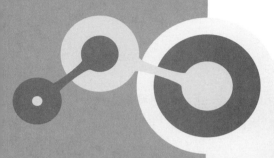

13

Referencing

Learning Outcomes

Upon completion of this laboratory chapter, you will be able to:

L-13-1   Differentiate between primary, secondary, and tertiary literature.

L-13-2   Explain the importance of maintaining a library in a pharmacy.

L-13-3   Compare and contrast the components of various reference books.

L-13-4   Define the meaning of the terms found in a drug monograph.

L-13-5   Identify the appropriate reference books for a particular setting.

L-13-6   Discover the use of the Internet in obtaining information affecting the pharmacy practice.

L-13-7   Identify various pharmacy Internet sites and the information they contain.

L-13-8   Understand the application of technology in obtaining pharmacy information.

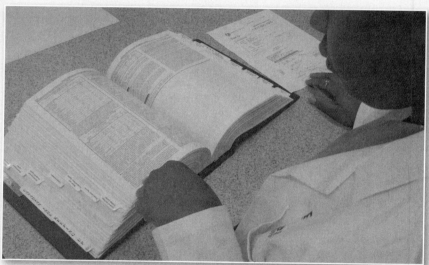

PTCB

In preparation for the certification examination, you should understand and perform activities associated with the following PTCB Knowledge Statement:

Domain I.   Assisting the Pharmacist in Serving Patients

Knowledge of drug information sources including printed and electronic reference materials (15)

Introduction to Referencing (L-13-2)

In 1975, the Millis Report was released and defined pharmacy as a knowledge-based profession and emphasized the role of the pharmacist in sharing knowledge about medications. State Boards of Pharmacy require that all pharmacies maintain a professional library appropriate for that particular practice, but must include the USP–NF and the Federal and State Controlled Substance Acts. From time to time, a pharmacy technician may be required to look up information for the pharmacist when counseling a patient or providing pharmacy information to a health care professional. It is extremely important that a pharmacy technician be knowledgeable in accessing information in the pharmacy.

Test Your Knowledge

Multiple Choice Questions

Answer the following multiple choice questions. When you have finished, check your answers and then review those areas that need improvement.

1. Which of the following reference books is updated monthly?(L-13-3)
   a. *Drug Facts and Comparisons*
   b. *Drug Topics Red Book*
   c. *Physicians' Desk Reference*
   d. *United States Pharmacopeia*

2. Which of the following reference books does *not* contain drug identification sections?(L-13-3)
   a. *Drug Facts and Comparisons*
   b. *Red Book*
   c. *Physicians' Desk Reference*
   d. *United States Pharmacopeia*

3. Which of the following reference books is available in a set of three volumes?(L-13-3)
   a. *Drug Facts and Comparisons*
   b. *Red Book*
   c. *Physicians' Desk Reference*
   d. *United States Pharmacopeia Drug Information*

4. Which of the following reference books is more valuable to community pharmacy than institutional pharmacy?(L-13-3)
   a. *Drug Facts and Comparisons*
   b. *Red Book*

   c. *The Injectable Drug Handbook*
   d. *The Pediatric Drug Handbook*

5. Which of the following reference books is more valuable to institutional pharmacy than community pharmacy?(L-13-3)
   a. *Drug Facts and Comparisons*
   b. *Red Book*
   c. *The Injectable Drug Handbook*
   d. *The Pediatric Drug Handbook*

6. Which of the following reference books contains drug reimbursement information?(L-13-3)
   a. *Drug Facts and Comparisons*
   b. *Red Book*
   c. *The Injectable Drug Handbook*
   d. *The Pediatric Drug Handbook*

7. Which of the following reference books contains information on labeled and unlabeled uses of a medication?(L-13-3)
   a. *Red Book*
   b. *Physicians' Desk Reference*
   c. *United States Pharmacopeia*
   d. *United States Pharmacopeia Drug Information*

8. Which of the following reference books contains a comprehensive listing of formulary drugs, which includes indications and adverse reactions?[(L-13-3)]
   a. *American Hospital Formulary Service Drug Information*
   b. *Red Book*
   c. *Ident-A-Drug*
   d. *Injectable Drug Handbook*

9. Which of the following reference books contains the following abbreviations: AWP, NDC, OBC, DP, NCPDP, HRI, UPCV, and SRP?[(L-13-3)]
   a. *Drug Facts and Comparisons*
   b. *Red Book*
   c. *Physicians' Desk Reference*
   d. *United States Pharmacopeia*

10. Which of the following reference books contains information relevant to the practice of pharmacy in any setting in the United States?[(L-13-3)]
    a. *American Drug Index*
    b. *Goodman and Gilman's The Pharmacological Basis of Therapeutics*
    c. *Martindale's Extra Pharmacopia*
    d. *Remington's Pharmaceutical Sciences*

11. In which of the following would a pharmacy technician be able to obtain continuing education?[(L-13-1, 13-6)]
    a. *Drug Topics*
    b. *Pharmacy Times*
    c. *US Pharmacist*
    d. All of the above

12. Which of the following is another name for a generic drug?[(L-13-x)]
    a. Brand name
    b. Chemical name
    c. Nonproprietary drug
    d. Trade name

13. Which of the following databases allows a hospital to report medication errors and be used as a tool for quality assurance programs?[(L-13-4)]
    a. BIOSIS
    b. EMBASE
    c. MEDLINE
    d. MEDMARX

14. Which of the following databases would provide information on a drug's toxicity?[(L-13-6, 13-7)]
    a. Pharmaceutical News Index
    b. Pharmaprojects

15. What would you find under the description of a medication?[(L-13-4)]
    a. Brand name
    b. Chemical name
    c. Generic name
    d. OTC name

16. How many categories are found in the *PDR*?[(L-13-3)]
    a. Four
    b. Five
    c. Six
    d. Seven

17. What pharmacy setting would benefit the most by maintaining a copy of USP <797> in its library?[(L-13-5)]
    a. Home health care
    b. Hospital pharmacy
    c. Mail-order pharmacy
    d. Retail pharmacy

18. In which of the following references would you find Japanese Accepted Names?[(L-13-3)]
    a. *USP-DI* Volume 3
    b. *USP Dictionary of USAN and International Drug Names*
    c. *USP–NF*
    d. All of the above

19. Who develops a formulary for an institution?[(L-13-5)]
    a. Institutional administrators
    b. Pharmacists
    c. Physicians
    d. P&T Committee

20. A parent informs the pharmacy that she has, found medication in her child's room and wants to know what it is. Which reference book might you use to identify the drug?[(L-13-3)]
    a. *AHFS Drug Information*
    b. *Goodman & Gillman's The Pharmacological Basis of Therapeutics*
    c. *Ident-A-Drug*
    d. *Remington's Pharmaceutical Sciences*

21. Which of the following reference books would be extremely beneficial if you are working in a pediatric hospital in the United States?[(L-13-3)]
    a. *American Drug Index*
    b. *Martindale's*
    c. *Neofax*
    d. *Red Book*

c. SEDBASE
d. TOXLIT

22. Which of the following is software to be used on a PDA by health care professionals?(L-13-8)
    a. Epocrates
    b. Hippocrates
    c. Socrates
    d. All of the above

23. As a pharmacy technician, you may be required to maintain your competency through continuing education. Which of the following organizations approves pharmacy continuing education programs?(L-13-6)
    a. ABHES
    b. ACPE
    c. ASCENT
    d. Pharm TEC

24. Which pharmacy magazine focuses an entire edition each month on a specific topic?(L-13-3)
    a. *Drug Topics*
    b. *Pharmacy Times*
    c. *RxTimes*
    d. *U.S. Pharmacist*

25. Which online pharmacy source works in conjunction with the National Institutes of Health?(L-13-7)
    a. EMBASE
    b. Medline Plus
    c. MedWatch
    d. Ovid

Identification

Print the meaning of the following terms, which are found in a monograph.

1. Indication(L-13-4)
   _____
   _____

2. Contraindication(L-13-4)
   _____
   _____

3. Description(L-13-4)
   _____
   _____

4. Clinical pharmacology(L-13-4)
   _____
   _____

5. Precautions(L-13-4)
   _____
   _____

6. Adverse reactions(L-13-4)
   _____
   _____

7. Overdosage(L-13-4)
   _____
   _____

8. Dosage and administration(L-13-4)
   _____
   _____

9. How supplied(L-13-4)
   _____
   _____

10. Clinical trials(L-13-4)
    _____
    _____

Acronyms

Print the meaning of the following acronyms.(L-13-4, 13-5)

ACPE _____
AERS _____
AWP _____
CEU(L-13-4) _____
CBER(L-13-5) _____

CDER _____
DP _____
NCPDP _____
NDC _____
NIH _____

OBC   _____

PDA   _____

PDR   _____

SRP   _____

USP–NF   _____

USPDI   _____

VAERS   _____

Apply Your Knowledge

1. The pharmacist asks you to look up information on a particular drug. Your pharmacy maintains a current edition of both the *PDR* and *Drug Facts and Comparisons*. Which book would you use and why?(L-13-3)

_____

_____

2. A patient brings in a prescription for Keflex 500 mg. In the patient's profile, it states that the patient is allergic to penicillin. Is there a problem with the patient receiving Keflex? If yes, what is the problem and what should be done?(L-13-2, 13-4)

_____

_____

3. A young female brings in a prescription for E.E.S. 400 mg. In the patient's profile, you notice that she is taking Triphasil 28. Is there a problem with the patient taking both of these medications? If so, what is the problem and how should it be resolved?(L-13-2, 13-4)

_____

_____

4. It is December 31 and a young man brings in a prescription for 56 tablets of Flagyl 250 mg. He asks if he can drink while taking the medication. What do you tell him and why?(L-13-2, 13-4)

_____

_____

5. A patient brings in a prescription for naproxen 500 mg for pain from Dr. A. J. Shedlock. This patient is receiving Nexium from another physician? Is there a problem and, if so, what is it?(L-13-2, 13-4)

_____

_____

6. You have been asked to compound a prescription for a suspension but you have forgotten how to do it. What reference book would you use and why?(L-13-5)

_____

_____

7. You are working in a hospital pharmacy and have been asked to prepare an IV of Drug X. What reference book would you use to verify that an incompatibility does occur between the drug and the intravenous solution that is chosen?(L-13-5)

_____

_____

8. As a certified pharmacy technician, you are required to obtain 20 CEUs every 2 years. How would you obtain these CEUs? Why did you choose this method?(L-13-2, 13-6)

_____

_____

9. What pregnancy code is assigned to a medication that has demonstrated evidence of fetal abnormalities?(L-13-4)

_____

_____

10. What is the advantage of using *Ident-A-Drug*?(L-13-5)

_____

_____

Practice Your Knowledge

Materials Needed

1. *PDR* or *Drug Facts and Comparisons*

Goal

To familiarize the pharmacy technician with using the either the *PDR* or *Drug Facts and* *Comparisons* in obtaining specific information on a medication.[(L-13-3)]

Assignment

Use the *PDR* or *Drug Facts and Comparisons* to collect information for the following medications:[(L-13-3)]

Drug Name and Strength	NDC Number	Drug Manufacturer	Recommended Daily Dose	Warnings
Humulin N Insulin 10 mL				
Novolin 70/30 Insulin 10 mL				
Zithromax Z-pak				
Lipitor 10 mg 100 tablets				
Serevent Inhaler				
Depakote 500 mg 100 tablets				
Mysoline 250 mg 100 tablets				
Tessalon Perles				
Diflucan 100 mg 100 tablets				
Sinemet 25/250 100 tablets				
Flonase Inhaler 14.2 mL				
Lidex Cream 15 g				
Coumadin 5 mg 100 tablets				
Eskalith 300 mg 100 capsules				
Dilantin 100 mg 1000 kapseals				
Glucophage 850 mg 100 tablets				
Proventil Inhaler 17 g				
Percodan 100 tablets				
Efudex Cream				
Micronase 5 mg 100 tablets				
Coreg 6.25 mg 100 tablets				
Wellbutrin XL 150 mg 30 tablets				

Calculation Corner

As a pharmacy technician, you may encounter a situation where you are required to prepare a compound for a prescription. Consider the following scenario.

A patient brings in this prescription:[L-13-5]

Dr. Joshua Stephenson

4500 Wisconsin Ave.

Washington, DC 20009

202-687-0300

Bruce Caldwell   March 28, 2010

1121 Arlington Blvd., Apt #324   Arlington, VA 22209

Coal Tar	2 g
Precipitated Sulfur	3 g
Salicylic Acid	1 g
Lidex Ointment	24 g
Aquabase	70 g

Apply once a day to the affected area

                                                                    Dr. Joshua Stephenson

Refill: 3 times in 6 months

What is the total weight of this compound? _____ [L-13-5]

Work Out the Solution

Pharm Facts—Research

Use the *PDR* or *Drug Facts and Comparison to* collect information for the cardiovascular medications listed in Table 13-1.[L-13-3]

Table 13-1

Brand Name	Generic Name	Strengths	Dosage Forms	Indications	Contraindications	Adverse Effects
Accupril						
Aldomet						
Avapro						
Calan						
Capoten						
Cardizem LA						
Coreg						
Corgard						
Coumadin						
Cozaar						
Crestor						
Diovan						
Hytrin						
Hyzaar						
Inderal						
Lanoxin						
Lescol						
Lipitor						
Lopid						
Lopressor						
Lotrel						
Lovenox						
Mephyton						
Mevacor						
Minipress						
Norpace						
Norvasc						
Persantine						
Plavix						
Pravachol						
Procardia						
Tenormin						
Trental						
Vaseretic						
Vasotec						
Zestril						
Zetia						
Zocor						

Did You Know?

An initiative has been proposed that by 2010 all prescriptions will be required to be submitted electronically.[L-13-7]

Practice Settings

14

Retail Setting

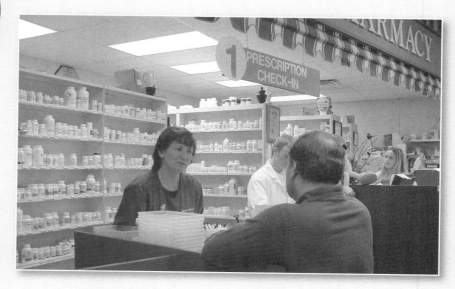

Learning Outcomes

Upon completion of this laboratory chapter, you will be able to:

L-14-1 Describe the layout of a retail pharmacy.

L-14-2 List the different types of retail pharmacies.

L-14-3 List the components of a prescription.

L-14-4 List information needed to fill a prescription.

L-14-5 Describe how to process a prescription.

L-14-6 Understand the connection between retail pharmacy and customer service.

L-14-7 Explain the various reasons why a prescription may be rejected by a third-party payer.

L-14-8 Understand how to find insurance information from the insurance card.

L-14-9 Describe the importance of the "flow of service."

(Continued)

PTCB

In preparation for the certification examination, you should understand and perform activities associated with the following PTCB Knowledge Statements:

Domain I. Assisting the Pharmacist in Serving Patients

Knowledge of pharmaceutical and medical abbreviations and terminology (4)

Knowledge of generic and brand names of pharmaceuticals (5)

Knowledge of information to be obtained from patient/patient's representative (21)

Knowledge of non-prescription (over-the-counter) formulations (28)

Knowledge of packaging requirements (33)

Knowledge of NDC number components (34)

Knowledge of information for prescription or medication order labels (36)

Knowledge of requirements regarding auxiliary labels (37)

Knowledge of requirements regarding patient package inserts (38)

Knowledge of quality improvement methods. (49)

Knowledge of pharmacy-related computer software for documenting the dispensing of prescriptions or prescriptions or medication orders (69)

Knowledge of reimbursement policies and plans (75)

Knowledge of legal requirements for pharmacist counseling of patient/ patient's representative (76)

Domain II. Maintaining Medication and Inventory Control Systems

Knowledge of formulary or approved stock list (5)

Knowledge of products used in packaging and repackaging (12)

Domain III. Participation in the Administration and Management of Pharmacy Practice

Knowledge of roles and responsibilities of pharmacists, pharmacy technicians, and other pharmacy employees (7)

Knowledge of legal and regulatory requirements for personnel, facilities, equipment, and supplies (8)

Knowledge of state board of pharmacy regulations (11)

Knowledge of sanitation requirements (19)

Knowledge of manual and computer-based systems for storing, receiving, and using pharmacy-related information (26)

Learning Outcomes   *(Cont'd)*

L-14-10 Identify the various categories of OTC medications found in a retail pharmacy.

L-14-11 Define the role of the pharmacy technician and the duties assigned to him or her in a retail pharmacy.

L-14-12 Explain the importance of the pharmacy's computer system.

Introduction to the Retail Setting(L-14-2)

Every day people take their prescriptions to be filled at the neighborhood drugstore, whether it is a chain drugstore, an independent drugstore a supermarket, or a mass merchandiser. According to the National Association of Drug Store Chains, in 2008, there were 3.5 billion prescriptions filled in the United States with retail sales of more than $253 billion. As you can see from these numbers, retail pharmacy is very much alive and growing. Retail pharmacy needs both knowledgeable and dependable pharmacy technicians to assist the pharmacist in filling prescriptions. Retail pharmacy allows pharmacy technicians to use their knowledge and skills every day to provide the correct drug with the correct strength and dosage form to be taken properly at the correct time by the correct patient. Pharmacy technicians play an integral part in the health care delivery system in the United States.

Test Your Knowledge

Multiple Choice Questions

Answer the following multiple choice questions. When you have finished, check your answers and then review those areas that need improvement.

1. What type of community pharmacy is CVS or Walgreens?(L-14-2)
   a. Chain pharmacy
   b. Franchise pharmacy
   c. Outpatient pharmacy
   d. Independently owned pharmacy

2. Who issues a permit for a retail pharmacy?(L-14-2)
   a. DEA
   b. FDA
   c. NABP
   d. State Board of Pharmacy

3. Which of the following pharmacy law needs to be adhered to in a retail pharmacy (may select more than one)?(L-14-2)
   a. Comprehensive Drug Abuse Prevention and Control Act of 1970
   b. OBRA-90
   c. HIPAA-1996
   d. All of the above

4. A physician has approved the use of a generic drug for a patient. What DAW code must be assigned for that prescription?(L-14-5)
   a. DAW 0
   b. DAW 1
   c. DAW 2
   d. DAW 4

5. Which of the following terms refers to the instructions to the patient?(L-14-3)
   a. Inscription
   b. Signa
   c. Signature
   d. Subscription

6. What DAW code would be assigned the following prescription?(L-14-5)

   Coumadin 5 mg   #30   Brand Name
                            Medically Necessary

   i tab po qd
   Ref × 5
   a. DAW 0
   b. DAW 1
   c. DAW 2
   d. DAW 3

7. Which of the following would be a correct DEA number for Dr. Shedlock?(L-14-3)
   a. AS1357921
   b. BS2468135
   c. FS3692464
   d. MS9876543

8. Which of the following is an example of an auxiliary label (may select more than one)?(L-14-5)
   a. May Cause Drowsiness
   b. Take on an Empty Stomach
   c. Take with Food
   d. All of the above

9. Which of the following terms refers to a predetermined amount of money or percentage of the cost that a patient will pay for a prescription?(L-14-5)
   a. Co-pay
   b. Deductible
   c. Fee for service
   d. Premium

10. A physician has approved the dispensing of a generic drug but the patient insists on receiving the brand name. What DAW code should be assigned to the prescription?(L-14-5)
    a. DAW 0
    b. DAW 1
    c. DAW 2
    d. DAW 4

11. Which pharmacy laws must be followed in retail pharmacy?(L-14-2)
    a. Federal laws
    b. Local laws
    c. State laws
    d. All of the above

12. Which of the following tasks cannot be performed by a pharmacy technician?(L-14-11)
    a. Counsel patients
    b. Count medication
    c. Input patient information into the computer system
    d. Order medications

13. Which of the following terms tells the pharmacy technician or pharmacist whether a refill is permitted by the physician?(L-14-3)
    a. DEA number
    b. Inscription
    c. Signa
    d. Subscription

14. If the directions "1–2 tab po q6–8 hours" appear on a prescription, how many days will 60 tablets last?(L-14-5)
    a. 7 days
    b. 10 days
    c. 15 days
    d. 20 days

15. Using the NDC number 12345-6789-01, which of the numbers identify the drug product?(L-14-4)
    a. 12345
    b. 6789
    c. 01
    d. 12345-6789-01

True/False

Mark True or False for each statement. If it is false, correct the statement to make it true.

1. _____ The inscription of a prescription includes the name of the medication, the strength, and the quantity.[(L-14-3)]

2. _____ The signa bid on a prescription means for the pharmacist to take this drug three times a day.[(L-14-3)]

3. _____ The Rx symbol on a prescription tells the pharmacist or pharmacy technician the correct directions to be included on the prescription.[(L-14-3)]

4. _____ If there are no refills indicated on a prescription by a physician, you may not refill the prescription without first obtaining permission from the physician's office.[(L-14-4, 14-5)]

5. _____ A physician assistant or a nurse practitioner may have the authority to write prescriptions for controlled and noncontrolled medications depending on state regulations.[(L-14-4)]

6. _____ A prescription with "prn" refills means the patient may have the prescription refilled at any time.[(L-14-3)]

7. _____ A pharmacy technician cannot accept a new prescription over the telephone from the physician's office.[(L-14-11)]

8. _____ A pharmacy technician cannot accept a faxed prescription from a physician's office.[(L-14-11)]

9. _____ A prescription must be maintained for a minimum of 2 years.[(L-14-5)]

10. _____ A faxed prescription is an example of e-prescribing.[(L-14-5)]

Matching

Match the abbreviation with its meaning.[(L-14-3, 14-4)]

_____ 1. am	A. twice a day
_____ 2. bid	B. afternoon/evening
_____ 3. elix	C. every 6 hours
_____ 4. g	D. bedtime
_____ 5. hs	E. by rectum
_____ 6. mL	F. as needed
_____ 7. pm	G. solution
_____ 8. po	H. morning
_____ 9. pr	I. by mouth
_____10. prn	J. milliliter
_____11. qid	K. gram
_____12. q6h	L. four times a day
_____13. sol	M. elixir
_____14. stat	N. syrup
_____15. supp	O. tablespoon
_____16. syr	P. three times a day
_____17. tbsp	Q. teaspoon
_____18. tid	R. vagina
_____19. tsp	S. suppository
_____20. vag	T. immediately

Acronyms

Print the meaning of the following acronyms.(L-13-4, 13-5)

CMS	_____	MAC	_____
CPOE	_____	NDC	_____
DAW	_____	NPI	_____
DEA	_____	OBRA	_____
DUE	_____	OTC	_____
HIPAA	_____	PBM	_____
HMO	_____	PPO	_____
IPA	_____		

Apply Your Knowledge

1. A prescription is rejected by a third-party payer with the following explanation "NDC Not Covered." How would you resolve this problem?(L-14-7)

_____

_____

2. A physician writes a prescription for a 90-day supply of a maintenance medication. The patient's prescription plan allows for a 30-day supply of medication. How would you explain to the patient why he or she only received a 30-day supply and what are the options to fill the prescription?(L-14-7)

_____

_____

3. A patient has been receiving the following prescription:

_____

_____

Dr. John Williams
1100 Wilson Blvd.
Arlington, VA 22209
703-527-1111

Ed Tarboosch
Hydrochlorothiazide 50 mg   #30
I po q am
Refill prn

                              Dr. John Williams

The prescription was written and filled initially on December 2, 2010. The patient attempts to refill the prescription on January 3, 2012, and the computer informs you that the prescription does not have any refills remaining and the prescription has expired. The patient tells you that his physician told him that he will need to take the medication the rest of his life. How would you handle this situation?(L-14-3, 14-12)

_____

_____

4. You are processing a prescription and receive a warning message during the Drug Utilization Evaluation step. What do you do?(L-14-5)

_____

_____

5. If you were filling a new prescription, would you fill it at a chain pharmacy, independent pharmacy, mass merchandiser, or grocery store? Why?(L-14-2)

_____

_____

6. Many retail pharmacies have drive-in windows to drop off and pick up prescriptions. What advantages and disadvantages do you find for drive-in windows?(L-14-1)

_____

_____

7. What can a pharmacy technician do to help eliminate rejections of prescriptions by third-party insurance providers?[L-14-4, 14-6, 14-7]

_____

_____

8. Explain the importance of collecting accurate patient information to be included in the patient's profile.[L-14-6]

_____

_____

9. What are the advantages and disadvantages of requiring prescription insurance cards to follow a standardized format?[L-14-8]

_____

_____

10. Should pharmacy technicians be able to counsel patients? Why or why not?[L-14-11]

_____

_____

Practice Your Knowledge

Materials Needed

1. Paper
2. Pen or pencil

Goal

To become familiar with the various OTC drug products that can be purchased at a retail pharmacy.[L-14-10]

Assignment

Visit a local retail pharmacy, select one product from each of the following drug OTC classifications, and complete the following table.[L-14-10]

Drug Classification	OTC Product	Active Ingredients	Dosage Form	Drug Interactions	Warnings
Analgesic					
Antidiarrheal agent					
Antifungal agent					
Antiseptic agent					
Carminative					
Contact lens agent					
Cough suppressant					
Dietary supplement					
Disinfectant					
Expectorant					
First aid agent					
Laxative					
Local anesthetic					
Nonsteroidal anti-inflammatory agent					
Nutritional supplement					
Stool softener					
Topical analgesic					
Topical antibiotic					
Vitamin					

Calculation Corner

A patient receives the following prescription:

> Cephalexin 500 mg   #40
> i cap po qid

Work Out the Solution

How many days will the prescription last the patient?_____ (L-14-5)

Pharm Facts—Research

Use the *PDR* or *Drug Facts and Comparisons* to complete Table 14-1. (L-14-1, 14-6)

Table 14-1

Brand Name	Generic Name	Indication	List Five Side Effects	Is the Medication a Controlled Substance?
Advair Diskus				
Ambien				
Amoxil				
Coumadin				
Fosamax				
Lasix				
Lexapro				
Lipitor				
Nexium				
Norvasc				
Prevacid				
Protonix				
Singular				
Synthroid				
Toprol XL				
Vicodin				
Zestril				
Zithromax				
Zoloft				
Zyrtec				

Did You Know?

According to the National Association of Drug Store Chains

- In 2007, there were 22,029 chain drugstores, 16,888 independent drugstores, 9,287 supermarkets, and 7,662 mass merchants that dispensed prescriptions.[L-14-2]
- In 2008, retail prescription sales totaled $253.6 billion, which is up 1.8% from $249.2 billion in 2007.[L-14-2]
- In 2008, retail pharmacies filled 3.5 billion prescriptions, which is up 0.6% from 3.52 billion in 2007.[L-14-2]
- In 2008, traditional chains filled 1.6 billion prescriptions, mass merchandisers filled 400 million prescriptions, supermarkets filled 481 million prescriptions, independent pharmacies filled 769 million prescriptions, and mail-order pharmacies filled 238 million prescriptions.[L-14-2] The average prescription price was $71.69 in 2008 versus $68.77 in 2007.[L-14-2]
- The average brand-name drug was $137.90 in 2008 compared to $121.18 in 2007.[L-14-2]
- The average generic price was $35.22 in 2008 versus $32.60 in 2007.[L-14-2]

15 Hospital/Inpatient Setting

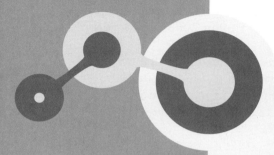

Learning Outcomes

Upon completion of this laboratory chapter, you will be able to:

L-15-1 Describe the hospital or inpatient setting.

L-15-2 Classify inpatient settings.

L-15-3 Identify organizations that regulate inpatient facilities.

L-15-4 Describe the policy and procedures manual.

L-15-5 Define *protocol* as it pertains to inpatient settings.

L-15-6 Define *formulary*.

L-15-7 Identify three types of medication orders.

L-15-8 Describe the role of the inpatient pharmacy technician.

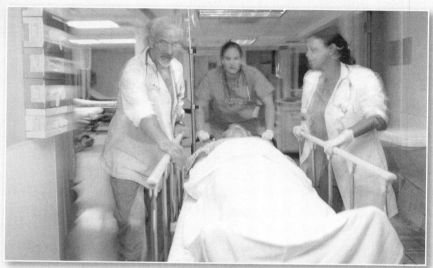

PTCB

In preparation for the certification examination, you should understand and perform activities associated with the following PTCB Knowledge Statement:

Domain I. Assisting the Pharmacist in Serving Patients

Knowledge of delivery system for distributing medications (43)

Knowledge of quality improvement methods (49)

Knowledge of infection control procedures (69)

Introduction to Hospital/Inpatient Setting(L-15-1, 15-2)

Hospitals (also known as inpatient facilities) require extensive pharmacy services as patients receiving care remain overnight in the facility. All medications, regardless of route of administration or prescription status, must be documented and reconciled. Pharmacy technicians, as a result, have many duties and responsibilities in an inpatient pharmacy setting. Because there are different types of facilities, there are also different types of pharmacy systems at work in hospitals to provide better service. Obviously, the inpatient pharmacy technician must be an integral part of the health care team to facilitate the provision of quality health care to patients. These laboratory activities will reinforce the concepts discussed in the corresponding textbook chapter.

Test Your Knowledge

Multiple Choice Questions

Answer the following multiple choice questions. When you have finished, check your answers and then review those areas that need improvement.

1. Which of the following agencies has no jurisdiction over inpatient pharmacies?(L-15-3)
   a. TJC, formerly JCAHO
   b. BOP
   c. DEA
   d. PTCB

2. Which of the following is a method of prescription data entry by the prescriber?(L-15-6)
   a. CPOE
   b. IV admixture
   c. TPN
   d. IVP

3. Which of the following is a means of administering a single packaged dose of medication?(L-15-1)
   a. IV piggyback
   b. Unit-dose
   c. Stock medications
   d. None of the above

4. Which of the following is a list of medications available for use in a facility?(L-15-5)
   a. Protocol
   b. Formulary
   c. Patient medication profile
   d. None of the above

5. Which of the following is *not* an acceptable medication order?(L-15-1)
   a. Verbal order
   b. Written order
   c. Electronic order
   d. All of the above are acceptable

6. Which of the following types of orders is used to indicate that the medication is needed immediately?(L-15-1)
   a. PRN order
   b. STAT order
   c. Reference order
   d. NPO order

7. Which of the following is responsible for establishing and updating the hospital formulary?(L-15-5)
   a. Pharmacy Services Department
   b. Pharmacy and Therapeutics Committee
   c. Board of directors
   d. Board of pharmacy

8. Which of the following organizations accredits hospitals?(L-15-3)
   a. NABP
   b. ASHP
   c. TJC, formerly JCAHO
   d. CDC

9. Therapeutic substitution involves(L-15-5)
   a. substituting the brand for the generic.
   b. substituting the most expensive drug for the least expensive drug.
   c. substituting a drug from a different category.
   d. substituting a drug from the same therapeutic class.

10. A set of guidelines and standards governing procedures or medication administration in a facility is a(L-15-4)
   a. formulary.
   b. medication administration record.
   c. protocol.
   d. policy and procedure manual.

11. According to TJC's (formerly JCAHO's) "Do Not Use" list, which of the following should be written to indicate that a medication is to be administered once a day?(L-15-6)
   a. QD
   b. qd
   c. daily
   d. qod

12. Which is *not* included in a patient's medication profile?(L-15-5)
   a. Laboratory test results
   b. Allergies
   c. Drugs dispensed
   d. Social Security number

13. What type of order is used to indicate that a patient receives medication as needed?(L-15-1, 15-5)
   a. Verbal order
   b. Prn order
   c. Stat order
   d. Electronic order

14. An inpatient facility has a single large pharmacy that serves all areas of the medical center. This is called a _____ (L-15-2)
   a. centralized model.
   b. decentralized model.
   c. noncomputerized model.
   d. none of the above.

15. Which of the following is *not* a responsibility of the inpatient pharmacy technician?(L-15-6)
   a. Medication administration
   b. Medication delivery and distribution
   c. Inventory management
   d. Crash cart inspection

16. If a pharmacy technician is allergic to latex gloves(L-15-6)
   a. the technician should use hypo allergenic gloves.
   b. the technician does not need to wear gloves.
   c. the technician cannot perform sterile compounding.
   d. none of the above.

17. Which of the following is *not* one of the "rights"?(L-15-3)
   a. Right drug
   b. Right dose
   c. Right technician
   d. Right route

18. Which of the following is *not* included on the medication label?(L-15-6)
   a. Patient's name
   b. Location information
   c. Dosage regimen
   d. Insurance coverage

19. A pharmacy system involving multiple pharmacies serving various areas in a facility is a(L-15-2)
   a. centralized system.
   b. decentralized system.
   c. computerized system.
   d. automated system.

20. Which of the following is a set of enforceable regulations governing compounding?(L-15-3)
   a. CPOE
   b. USP <797>
   c. CDC
   d. DEA

21. All of the following are common aspects of community hospitals *except*(L-15-2)
   a. has more than 500 patient beds.
   b. has limited resources for emergency care.
   c. has limited resources for surgery.
   d. is small, relative to a teaching hospital.

22. Inpatient facility standards are enforced by all of the following *except*(L-15-3)
   a. CMS.
   b. TJC, formerly JCAHO.
   c. FDA.
   d. BOP.

23. The steps or methods by which the regulations of an inpatient facility are carried out are called[L-15-4]
    a. rules.
    b. policies.
    c. procedures.
    d. standards.

24. According to TJC's (formerly JCAHO's) "Do Not Use" list, a zero should[L-15-3]
    a. be included before the decimal, as in 0.X mg.
    b. be included after the decimal, as in X.0 mg.
    c. always be used.
    d. never be used.

25. Which of the following agencies enforces standards relating to the safety of the workforce?[L-15-3]
    a. CMS
    b. OSHA
    c. BOP
    d. DEA

Matching[L-15-3]

Match the agency acronym with its area of jurisdiction

1. _____ CMS
2. _____ BOP
3. _____ OSHA
4. _____ TJC
5. _____ DEA

A. Accredits health care facilities
B. Enforces workplace safety regulations
C. Enforces pharmacy laws
D. Determines the capacity of the institution to provide care
E. Governs the use of controlled substances

Apply Your Knowledge

1. Describe restrictions in an area where hazardous drugs are stored.[L-15-1, 15-2]

    _____
    _____
    _____

2. List five responsibilities of the inpatient pharmacy technician.[L-15-6]

    _____
    _____
    _____

3. The use of electronic devices or robotics to process drug orders is called _____.[L-15-6]

4. A list of medications for use in a facility or by a health care plan determined by Pharmacy and Therapeutics Committee is called a(n) _____.[L-15-1]

5. Medications packaged as a single dose are termed _____.[L-15-1]

6. Who is ultimately responsible for the accuracy of dispensed medications?[L-15-6]

7. List at least five duties of an inpatient pharmacy technician.[L-15-6]

8. What is **OSHA** and what is its role?[L-15-3]

9. List at least three specialty tasks of inpatient pharmacy technicians.[L-15-6]

10. List the five rights of medication administration.[L-15-4]

Practice Your Knowledge

Materials Needed

1. Internet access
2. Poster board
3. Pens (of various colors)
4. Pencils (of various colors)
5. Paper

Goal

To evaluate the students' understanding of inpatient pharmacy practice settings in their local area.[(L-15-1, 15-2)]

Assignment

1. Identify all of the hospitals/medical centers within a 50-mile (or 100-mile, depending on your area) radius of your school. For large metropolitan areas, it may be necessary to evaluate the area in quadrants (north, south, east, west).[(L-15-1)]

2. Using the Internet, search for the Web sites of the facilities you identified as being in your area what type of facility each is (community hospital, large medical center, teaching or university hospital).[(L-15-2)]

3. Write down the specifics of the institutions along with contact information. Identify the type of pharmacy services that are provided in each facility.[(L-15-2)]

4. Print out a map of the area. Identify each type of facility using a different color of pen or pencil. [(L-15-1, 15-2)]

5. Go to your state pharmacy board's Web site and check the licensure status of the facilities' pharmacies.[(L-15-3)]

6. Go to TJC's Web site and check the accreditation status of the facilities you identified.[(L-15-3)]

7. Present your findings to the class. [(L-15-2, 15-3)]

Calculation Corner

You have just been hired to work in a hospital pharmacy, but your only experience in hospital pharmacy was during your externship in the pharmacy technician program. The supervising pharmacist understands your concerns, so he asks you to perform the following calculations:

1. How many grams of dextrose are contained in a 100-mL D5W bag? _____ [(L-15-6)]

2. How many grams of dextrose would be contained in a 500-mL D5W bag? _____ [(L-15-6)]

Work Out the Solution

LOT   EXP

5%   **2B0087**
                  NDC 0338-0017-48
**Dextrose
Injection USP**

100 mL SINGLE DOSE CONTAINER
EACH 100 mL CONTAINS
5 g DEXTROSE HYDROUS
USP pH 4.0 (3.2 TO 6.5) OSMOLARITY
252 mOsmol/L (CALC) STERILE
NONPYROGENIC READ PACKAGE INSERT FOR
FULL INFORMATION ADDITIVES MAY BE
INCOMPATIBLE DOSAGE INTRAVENOUSLY AS
DIRECTED BY A PHYSICIAN CAUTIONS MUST
NOT BE USED IN SERIES CONNECTIONS DO
NOT ADMINISTER SIMULTANEOUSLY WITH
BLOOD DO NOT USE UNLESS SOLUTION IS
CLEAR RX ONLY

VIAFLEX CONTAINER   PL 146 PLASTIC

BAXTER VIAFLEX AND PL 146 ARE
TRADEMARKS OF BAXTER INTERNATIONAL INC

Baxter
BAXTER HEALTHCARE CORPORATION
DEERFIELD IL 60015 USA
MADE IN USA

Baxter and Viaflex are registered trademarks of Baxter International Inc. Used with permission.

Pharm Facts—Research

Table 15-1 contains names of common agents used in inpatient settings. Complete the missing information. How much can you do from memory?[L-15-1]

Table 15-1

Brand Name	Generic Name	Therapeutic Classification	Dosage Forms
	midazolam		
	heparin		
	metoclopramide		
Rocephin			
Kytril			
	levothyroxine		
	enalaprilat		
Lopressor			
	vancomycin		

Did You Know?

The first hospital established in the thirteen colonies was Philadelphia Hospital in Pennsylvania in 1751. By late 1752, the hospital hired a "salaried apothecary" to prepare medications for the patients.[L-15-1]

Source: National Library of Medicine, **www.nlm.nih.gov/hmd/pdf/images.pdf.**

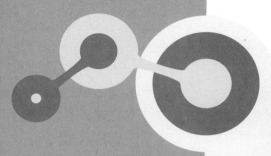

16

Other Environments

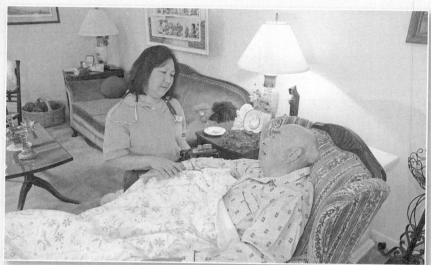

Learning Outcomes

Upon completion of this laboratory chapter, you will be able to:

L-16-1 Explain the need for pharmacy technicians in various settings in the practice of pharmacy.

L-16-2 Clarify the services made available to patients in these settings.

L-16-3 Describe the processing of prescriptions in the various settings.

L-16-4 Compare and contrast the unique characteristics of each of these settings.

L-16-5 Explain the function of Pharmacy Benefit Management (PBM) firms.

L-16-6 Identify the payment process in each of these situations.

L-16-7 Distinguish specific skills necessary to be successful in each of these settings.

(Continued)

PTCB

In preparation for the certification examination, you should understand and perform activities associated with the following PTCB Knowledge Statements:

Domain I. Assisting the Pharmacist in Serving Patients

Knowledge of federal, state, and/or practice site regulations, code of ethics, and standards pertaining to the practice of pharmacy (1)

Knowledge of therapeutic equivalence (6)

Knowledge of requirements for dispensing controlled substances (44)

Domain III. Participating in the Administration and Management of Pharmacy Practice

Knowledge of third-party reimbursement systems (31)

Introduction to Other Environments^(L-16-1)

Career opportunities for pharmacy technicians have increased enormously since 1995. These opportunities exist in many new and exciting pharmacy settings, many of which did not exist 10 years ago. Each of these settings requires special skills of the pharmacy technician. One common characteristic exists among all of them—the pharmacy technician assists the pharmacist in the practice of pharmacy. Pharmacy practice will continue to expand in the years to come with many new opportunities arising to meet the demands of a changing population.

Learning Outcomes *(Cont'd)*

L-16-8 Recognize specific legislation that affects a specific pharmacy environment..

L-16-9 Identify the role, responsibilities, and duties of both the pharmacist and pharmacy technician in different pharmacy settings.

Test Your Knowledge

Multiple Choice Questions

Answer the following multiple choice questions. When you have finished, check your answers and then review those areas that need improvement.

1. Which of the following is an example of a long-term care facility?^(L-16-2)
   a. Chronic disease hospitals
   b. Hospice care
   c. Nursing homes
   d. All of the above

2. What type of services may be provided to patients in a long-term care facility?^(L-16-3)
   a. Health care
   b. Personal care
   c. Social services
   d. All of the above

3. What term describes the submission of a prescription claim to an insurance provider?^(L-16-6)
   a. Adjudication
   b. Drug Utilization Evaluation
   c. Prescription screening
   d. Quality assurance check

4. Which form of pharmacy environment would perform pharmacy audits?^(L-16-2)
   a. Federal government
   b. Long-term care
   c. Mail-order pharmacy
   d. Managed-care pharmacy

5. Which of the following pharmacy settings would *not* prepare total parenteral nutrition?^(L-16-2, 16-3)
   a. Federal government
   b. Home infusion pharmacy
   c. Long-term care pharmacy
   d. Mail-order pharmacy

6. Which pharmacy setting may require a pharmacy technician to repackage and relabel medications?^(L-16-7, 19.9)
   a. Home infusion pharmacy
   b. Long-term pharmacy
   c. Nuclear pharmacy
   d. Pharmacy manufacturers

7. Which pharmacy setting uses radionucleotides?^(L-16-2)
   a. Home infusion pharmacy
   b. Long-term care pharmacy
   c. Managed-care pharmacy
   d. Nuclear pharmacy

8. Which of the following methods of administration are used for home infusion patients?^(L-16-2)
   a. Epidural
   b. Intravenous
   c. Subcutaneous
   d. All of the above

9. Which pharmacy setting requires a pharmacy to maintain a professional library?(L-16-4)
   a. Long-term care pharmacy
   b. Mail-order pharmacy
   c. Managed-care pharmacy
   d. All of the above

10. Which of the following is an advantage of a mail-order pharmacy?(L-16-2, L-16-4)
    a. Cost savings
    b. Larger variety of medications
    c. Patient convenience
    d. All of the above

11. Which of the following can be attributed to an increase in the need for a home infusion pharmacy?(L-16-1, L-16-2)
    a. Growth in an aging market
    b. Improvements in the quality of vascular lines
    c. Less expensive than patient hospitalization
    d. All of the above

12. Which pharmacy setting allows for the return and the reusing of medications (may select more than one)?(L-16-2, L-16-4)
    a. Home health care
    b. Long-term care pharmacy
    c. Managed-care pharmacy
    d. All of the above

13. Which of the following may a pharmacy technician perform in home infusion pharmacy?(L-16-7)
    a. Develop a formulary for an institution
    b. Prepare sterile medication orders
    c. Prepare unit-dose medications
    d. Replace emergency boxes

14. Who designs, administers, and manages a prescription drug benefit?(L-16-5)
    a. HMO
    b. IPA
    c. PBM
    d. PPO

15. Which third-party program provides health benefits for the dependents of military personnel?(L-16-6)
    a. CHAMPVA
    b. Medicare
    c. TRICARE
    d. All of the above

16. Which part of Medicare pays for prescriptions in a retail setting?(L-16-6)
    a. Part A
    b. Part B

    c. Part C
    d. Part D

17. Which of the following is a method to control prescription costs in managed care?(L-16-3)
    a. Day supply
    b. Drugs not covered
    c. Online adjudication
    d. All of the above

18. Which of the following might appear during drug utilization evaluation?(L-16-5, L-16-6)
    a. Contraindication
    b. Drug interaction
    c. Under- and overdosing
    d. All of the above

19. Which of the following is a goal of managed care?(L-16-2)
    a. High quality
    b. Lowest cost
    c. Reasonable access
    d. All of the above

20. Which of the following types of medications are prepared in a home infusion pharmacy?(L-16-2)
    a. Analgesics
    b. Antibiotics
    c. Total parenteral nutrition
    d. All of the above

21. Which pharmacy setting does *not* require performing a drug utilization evaluation?(L-16-2, 16-3)
    a. Home infusion
    b. Long-term care
    c. Mail order
    d. Pharmaceutical company

22. Which of the following explanations may be made for the rejection of a prescription insurance claim to a third-party provider?(L-16-2)
    a. Drug not covered
    b. Patient not covered
    c. Refill too soon
    d. All of the above

23. A long-term care pharmacy may accept the return and reuse prescription medication provided which of the following?(L-16-2, L-16-3)
    a. Medications are dispensed in tamper-resistant containers
    b. Returned medications are not controlled substances

c. System is in place to track the reuse of all medications

d. All of the above

24. Which of the following is *not* a task a pharmacy technician would perform in a long-term care pharmacy?(L-16-7)

a. Prepare compounded medications

b. Prepare, package, and label medications for residents in a long-term care facility

c. Prepare radionucleotides

d. Replace emergency boxes when needed

25. Which of the following documents must be signed by a physician for home infusion medications?(L-16-2, L-16-9)

a. Certificate of Medical Necessity and Plan of Treatment

b. Certificate of Responsibility

c. DNR

d. Physician's Directive

True/False

Mark True or False for each statement. If it is false, correct the statement to make it true.

1. _____The use of an emergency drug does not require a physician's order.(L-16-2, 16-3)

2. _____Drug Utilization Evaluation (DUE) is not required to be performed in a long-term care pharmacy.(L-16-2, 16-4)

3. _____Medication dispensed to long-term care facilities may use a unit-dose system.(L-16-2)

4. _____VIPPS is used to monitor medications a patient receives in a long-term care facility.(L-16-2)

5. _____Pharmacy technicians perform injections on patients in home infusion pharmacy.(L-16-7)

6. _____Pharmacy technicians monitor a patient's IV therapy.(L-16-7)

7. _____Bar coding may be used as part of quality assurance in mail-order pharmacy.(L-16-2)

8. _____A pharmaceutical sales or detail-person provides information regarding medications to pharmacies only.(L-16-2)

9. _____The pharmacist is not required to counsel patients in a mail-order pharmacy.(L-16-2, 16-3)

10. _____Pharmacy technicians working in a nuclear pharmacy do not require additional knowledge or training.(L-16-7)

11. _____Radiation safety is a component of home infusion pharmacy.(L-16-2)

12. _____Members of the military wishing to become pharmacy technicians undergo an approved pharmacy technician program developed by the ASHP.(L-16-1)

13. _____Radiopharmaceuticals are prepared in home infusion pharmacy.(L-16-2)

14. _____A long-term care pharmacy is always located in a long-term care facility.(L-16-2)

15. _____A faxed Schedule II medication to a long-term care pharmacy does not require a handwritten prescription from the prescribing physician.(L-16-2, 16-9)

Acronyms

Print the meaning of the following acronyms.(L-16-2)

ASHP _____

CDC _____

DHS _____

DME _____

DUE _____

HIS _____

HMO _____

IPA _____

IV _____

MCO _____

NABP _____   PPO _____
NIH _____   TJC _____
P&T _____   VIPPS _____
PBM _____

Apply Your Knowledge

1. In most situations, managed-care organizations will reimburse a retail pharmacy only for a 30-day supply of a medication. How would you handle a patient who presents you with a prescription for a 90-day supply of medication and three refills? What would you say to the patient if he or she questions receiving only a 30-day supply?(L-16-3)

_____
_____

2. Which type of pharmacy practice interests you the most and why?(L-16-2)

_____
_____

3. What special skills are necessary for a pharmacy technician to practice in a home infusion pharmacy?(L-16-7, 16-9)

_____
_____

4. Identify 5 long-term care facilities in your community and find out who provides medications for their patients.(L-16-2, 16-3)

_____
_____

5. Are technical or interpersonal skills more important for someone who is working for a pharmacy manufacturer? Why?(L-16-7)

_____
_____

6. Identify and list 10 medications found in an emergency box or crash cart in a long-term care facility. Why would these medications be needed?(L-16-3)

_____
_____

7. Identify the roles of all the practitioners in preparing home infusion medications.(L-16-2, 16-3)

_____
_____

8. What are the advantages and disadvantages of managed care?(L-16-2)

_____
_____

9. Which type of co-payment (fixed or percentage) is best for the customer? For the pharmacy?(L-16-6)

_____
_____

10. Who benefits from a drug formulary—the patient, the pharmacy, or the PBM? Why?(L-16-8)

_____
_____

Practice Your Knowledge

Materials Needed

1. Paper
2. Pen or pencil
3. Internet access

Goal

To identify skills that are necessary for a pharmacy technician to be successful in a long-term pharmacy.(L-16-9)

Assignment

Visit **www.omnicare.com** and identify the various career opportunities available for pharmacy technicians. What is the role of the pharmacy technician in each of these positions? Do you possess the necessary skills and knowledge to work in a long-term care pharmacy? If not, what areas should you focus on?

Calculation Corner

A physician orders 50 mL of D10W that contains ampicillin 1.25 million units. The IV is to be infused over 30 minutes.

1. How many units of ampicillin will the patient receive after 15 minutes? _____ (L-16-3)

Work Out the Solution

Pharm Facts—Research

Use the *PDR* or *Drug Facts and Comparisons* to complete Table 16-1.(L-16-3)

Table 16-1

Brand Name	Generic Name	Drug Classification	Dosage Forms	List Two Indications of the Medication	List Three Adverse Effects of the Medication
Advair					
Ambien					
Augmentin					
Avonex					
Biaxin					
Combivir					
Cordarone					
Detrol LA					
Dilantin					
Duragesic					
Efudex					
Focalin					

(Continued)

Table 16-1 *(Continued)*

Brand Name	Generic Name	Drug Classification	Dosage Forms	List Two Indications of the Medication	List Three Adverse Effects of the Medication
Imuran					
Lexapro					
Lovenox					
Lupron					
Maxalt-MLT					
Oxycontin					
Procrit					
Protonix					
Strattera					
Tegretol					
Wellbutrin					
Xopenex					

Using the drugs listed in the preceding exercise, in Table 16-2 list the types of pharmacies that may stock them for their patients.[L-16-2, 16-3]

Table 16-2

Brand Name	Retail Pharmacy	Hospital Pharmacy	Long-Term Care Pharmacy	Mail-Order Pharmacy	Federal Pharmacy
Advair					
Ambien					
Augmentin					
Avonex					
Biaxin					
Combivir					
Cordarone					
Detrol LA					
Dilantin					
Duragesic					
Efudex					
Focalin					
Imuran					
Lexapro					

Brand Name	Retail Pharmacy	Hospital Pharmacy	Long-Term Care Pharmacy	Mail-Order Pharmacy	Federal Pharmacy
Lovenox					
Lupron					
Maxalt-MLT					
Oxycontin					
Procrit					
Protonix					
Strattera					
Tegretol					
Wellbutrin					
Xopenex					

Did You Know?

Kaiser Permanente, one of the leading and oldest HMOs in the United States, was founded at the end of the Depression in California through the efforts of Dr. Sidney Garfield and Harold Hatch. Hatch proposed the idea that insurance companies pay a fixed amount per day per patient to the health care provider up-front. An individual was able to pay 5 cents a day for health care coverage under this plan. For an additional 5 cents the person would be able to obtain coverages for nonwork-related conditions. It is through the efforts of these two men that preventative health care was born.[L-16-2]

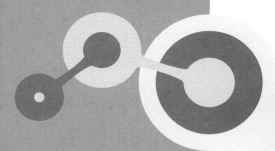

17

Inventory Management

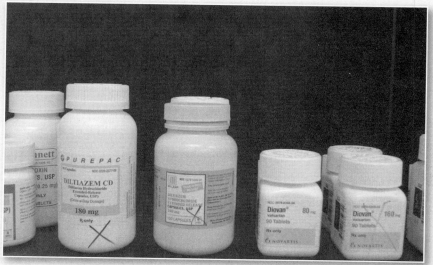

Learning Outcomes

Upon completion of this laboratory chapter, you will be able to:

L-17-1 Justify the importance of inventory management in the practice of pharmacy.

L-17-2 Discuss the principles of inventory management.

L-17-3 Give reasons for the importance of a formulary system in institutional pharmacy.

L-17-4 Describe the function of a group purchasing organization.

L-17-5 List the steps in ordering medication for the pharmacy.

L-17-6 Explain the processes in ordering of controlled substances.

L-17-7 Demonstrate the steps in receiving medication from a supplier.

L-17-8 Justify the importance of rotating stock upon receipt of new product.

(Continued)

PTCB

In preparation for the certification examination, you should understand and perform activities associated with the following PTCB Knowledge Statement:

Domain II. Maintaining Medication and Inventory Control Systems

Knowledge of drug product laws and regulations and professional standards related to obtaining medication supplies, durable medical equipment, and products (1)

Knowledge of pharmaceutical industry procedures for obtaining pharmaceuticals (2)

Knowledge of purchasing policies, procedures, and practices (3)

Knowledge of formulary and approved stock list (5)

Knowledge of PAR and reorder levels and drug usage (6)

Knowledge of inventory receiving process (7)

Knowledge of the DEA controlled substance ordering forms (9)

Knowledge of regulatory requirements regarding record keeping for repackaged products, recalled products, and refunded products (10)

Knowledge of policies, procedures, and practices for inventory procedures (11)

Knowledge of the FDA's classifications of recalls (14)

Knowledge of systems to identify and return expired and unsalable products (15)

Knowledge of rules and regulations for removal and disposal of products (16)

Knowledge of regulatory requirements and professional standards (18)

Knowledge of medication distribution and controlled systems for controlled substances, investigational drugs, and hazardous materials and wastes (23)

Knowledge of quality assurance policies, procedures, and practices for medication, and inventory control systems (25)

Learning Outcomes *(Cont'd)*

L-17-9 Describe the storage of medications in a pharmacy.

L-17-10 Calculate inventory turnover rate.

L-17-11 Explain the processes involved in the destruction of controlled substances.

L-17-12 Describe the importance and preparation of a yearly physical inventory.

L-17-13 Contrast the various types of inventories found in pharmacy practice.

L-17-14 Explain the handling of "unsaleable" merchandise.

L-17-15 Disclose the procedures involved with the development of new drug products.

L-17-16 Explain the methods in obtaining investigational new drug products.

L-17-17 Describe the drug recall process.

Introduction to Inventory Management(L-17-1)

An inventory is a listing of goods or items available for use in a normal business operation. One of the largest expenses in a pharmacy is its inventory. It is the responsibility of the pharmacist to ensure that the pharmacy stocks the correct medications of the proper dosage forms and strengths that are needed by their patients. A pharmacy, that maintains a proper inventory of medications provides excellent customer service to its customers.

Test Your Knowledge

Multiple Choice Questions

Answer the following multiple choice questions. When you have finished, check your answers and then review those areas that need improvement.

1. Which of the following is a source for obtaining medications for a pharmacy?(L-17-5)
   a. Company warehouse
   b. Drug manufacturer
   c. Drug wholesaler
   d. All of the above

2. Which DEA form is used to transfer Schedule II medications to another pharmacy?(L-17-6)
   a. DEA Form 41
   b. DEA Form 222
   c. DEA Form 224
   d. No DEA form is required

3. What type of inventory must be conducted every 2 years?[(L-17-13)]
   a. Biannual
   b. Biennial
   c. Initial
   d. Perpetual

4. Which of the statements is false?[(L-17-1)]
   a. Inventory management maximizes the costs associated with placing an order.
   b. Inventory management minimizes the costs associated with placing an order to a wholesaler.
   c. Inventory management provides for an adequate supply of product to be available to the customer.
   d. Inventory management reduces the carrying cost in drug products.

5. Which of the following should be checked on the invoice when receiving orders from a wholesaler?[(L-17-7)]
   a. Drug name
   b. Drug strength
   c. Quantity received
   d. All of the above

6. Why would a pharmacy establish a contract with a prime vendor?[(L-17-5)]
   a. Prime vendors maintain a very high in-stock position.
   b. Prime vendors provide competitive pricing.
   c. Prime vendors may provide both hardware and software to the pharmacy to maintain proper inventory levels.
   d. All of the above.

7. If you receive damaged medication from a wholesaler, when should it be notified?[(L-17-7)]
   a. Immediately
   b. Within a week
   c. Within the current billing cycle
   d. Within the fiscal year

8. What DEA form is used to order Schedule III–V drugs?[(L-17-6)]
   a. DEA Form 41
   b. DEA Form 222
   c. DEA Form 224
   d. No DEA form is required

9. Which of the following individuals or (organizations) may initiate a clinical investigation of an IND?[(L-17-15)]
   a. Academic institution
   b. Governmental agency

   c. Pharmaceutical company
   d. All of the above

10. What is the goal of a sponsor of an IND?[(L-17-15)]
    a. Determine the parameters of the proposed study
    b. Initiate and conduct the investigation
    c. Take responsibility for the administration or dispensing of the medication to the subjects in the study
    d. Submit data demonstrating that the proposed medication is safe to use in clinical studies

11. Which of the following is *not* a type of investigational new drug?[(L-17-15)]
    a. Emergency Use IND
    b. Investigator IND
    c. Prophylactic IND
    d. Treatment IND

12. Which phase during an IND investigation utilizes healthy individuals?[(L-17-15)]
    a. Phase I
    b. Phase II
    c. Phase III
    d. Phase IV

13. Who will establish policies and procedures regarding INDs in a hospital?[(L-17-16)]
    a. DEA
    b. FDA
    c. TJC, formerly JCAHO
    d. P&T Committee

14. Which type of drug recall is not likely to cause adverse health consequences?[(L-17-17)]
    a. Class I
    b. Class II
    c. Class III
    d. Class IV

15. What temperature classification does not exceed 8°C (46°F)?[(L-17-9)]
    a. Cold
    b. Cool
    c. Warm
    d. Excessive heat

16. What does a shorter turnaround time for orders allow?[(L-17-2)]
    a. Lower inventory stock turns
    b. More time and manpower needed for payment of invoices
    c. Smaller physical inventories
    d. All of the above

17. What term is used to indicate a pharmacy's ability to purchase contract items?(L-17-4)
    a. Bid
    b. Contract
    c. Velocity
    d. All of the above

18. Which of the following should be done in stocking pharmaceuticals?(L-17-7)
    a. Check the expiration date
    b. Reread the label several times
    c. Rotate stock
    d. All of the above

19. Which of the following is an advantage of just-in-time purchasing?(L-17-5)
    a. Fewer dollars invested in inventory
    b. Shorter turnaround times
    c. Smaller physical inventories
    d. All of the above

20. Which of the following will result in nonbid purchases?(L-17-4)
    a. Manufacturing back order
    b. Poor purchasing practices
    c. Wholesaler temporarily out of stock
    d. All of the above

True/False

Mark True or False for each statement. If it is false, correct the statement to make it true.

1. _____ When receiving an order from a drug manufacturer or your warehouse, it does not matter where the medication is placed on the shelf.(L-17-8)

2. _____ You should always rotate the medication on the shelf.(L-17-8)

3. _____ It is a good idea to place an X on the front of an opened container of medicine.(L-17-7, 17-8)

4. _____ There is no time limit in reporting a shortage on an order.(L-17-7)

5. _____ It is against the law for outdated medication to comingle with current medication.(L-17-14)

6. _____ A pharmacy registers with the DEA using DEA Form 226.(L-17-6)

7. _____ Therapeutic equivalent is the same as therapeutic interchange.(L-17-3)

8. _____ A blanket authorization for the destruction of controlled substances is valid only in pharmacies dispensing more than 200 prescriptions per day.(L-17-11)

9. _____ A light-resistant container protects the contents from the effects of light by virtue of the specific properties of the material of which it is composed, including any coating applied to it.(L-17-9)

10. _____ A drug recall involves the use of a lot number to identify a particular batch of the product.(L-17-17)

11. _____ It is extremely important for the pharmacy to respond to a drug recall even if it does not have any of the recalled medication in their pharmacy.(L-17-17)

12. _____ Recalled medication needs to be isolated from other medication in the pharmacy.(L-17-17)

13. _____ Medication that has tamper-evident packaging should be removed from the shelf if the seal has been broken.(L-17-14)

14. _____ A multiple-dose container is used for enteral medications.(L-17-9)

15. _____ A "want book" may be used in both retail and institutional pharmacies.(L-17-5)

16. _____ A "Warm Temperature" is any temperature between 30° and 40°C (86° to 104°F).(L-17-9)

17. _____ Group Purchasing Organizations (GPOs) purchase medications for institutions.(L-17-4)

18. _____ A contract compliance report is issued to show which bid items were not purchased and the amount of money lost by the institution.

19. _____ A long-term care facility may transfer controlled substances to a pharmacy.(L-17-6)

20. _____ A lot number is the same thing as a batch number.(L-17-17)

Apply Your Knowledge

1. Explain the impact of proper inventory management on customer service.[(L-17-1)]

   _____

   _____

2. What types of problems may develop as a result of failing to properly check an order from a vendor?[(L-17-7)]

   _____

   _____

3. What types of problems may develop if you fail to use the want book properly?[(L-17-5)]

   _____

   _____

4. What types of problems may result if you do not rotate products properly?[(L-17-8)]

   _____

   _____

5. What types of problems may develop if you do not separate outdated merchandise from the remaining merchandise in the pharmacy?[(L-17-14)]

   _____

   _____

6. Looking at the following Pharmacy Compliance Report. Which brand of morphine sulfate (1mg/mL) should the pharmacy order? How much money is saved by ordering this brand of morphine sulfate?[(L-17-4)]

   _____

   _____

Pharmacy Compliance Report

Drug Manufacturer	Brand Name	Package Size	Quantity	Unit Cost	Extended Cost	Savings
Baxter	Morphine Sulfate	10.00 mL	40	$ 6.89	$ 275.60	
ESI Lederle	Duramorph	10.00 mL	40	$ 1.27	$ 50.80	

7. How many inventory turns will a pharmacy have if the average inventory is $355,743 and the pharmacy has yearly sales of $5.2 million?[(L-17-10)]

   _____

   _____

8. You have been notified from drug manufacturer A that amoxicillin 500 mg in quantities of 1000 capsules with an expiration date of September 2012 and a lot number of X1075Z42 is being recalled because of a potency problem. What would you do?[(L-17-17)]

   _____

   _____

9. What advantage does just-in-time ordering provide the pharmacy?[(L-17-2, 17-5)]

   _____

   _____

10. Which is better for a pharmacy, maintaining a low inventory or a high inventory?[(L-17-1, 17-10)]

    _____

    _____

Practice Your Knowledge

Materials Needed

1. Pencil
2. Calculator

Goal

To demonstrate an understanding of maintaining a perpetual inventory.[(L-17-13)]

Assignment

Complete the perpetual inventory for Percocet using the following information:[L-17-13]

1. Invoice MGH 10061908 — June 19, 2010

   DEA Form 222 — 123456

   Percocet 5 — 5 × 100 tablets/bottle

2. June 19, 2010 — Rx 125678 — Dispensed 50 tablets
3. June 19, 2010 — Rx 125698 — Dispensed 25 tablets
4. June 20, 2010 — Rx 125789 — Dispensed 100 tablets
5. June 21, 2010 — Rx 125900 — Dispensed 30 tablets
6. June 23, 2010 — Rx 126335 — Dispensed 60 tablets
7. June 23, 2010 — Rx 126338 — Dispensed 20 tablets
8. June 23, 2010 — Rx 126380 — Dispensed 100 tablets
9. Invoice MGH 10062508 — June 25, 2008

   DEA Form 222 — 123457

   Percocet 5 — 5 × 100 tablets

10. June 26, 2010 — 124899 — Dispensed 100 tablets
11. June 27, 2010 — 125000 — Dispensed 10 tablets
12. June 27, 2010 — 125009 — Dispensed 20 tablets

Date	Prescription Number	Quantity Dispensed	Invoice Number	Quantity Received	Ending Inventory

Calculation Corner

Complete the following table to indicate the maximum number of bottles or containers you would order without exceeding the maximum quantity.[L-17-5]

Drug	Package Size	Qty on Hand	Max. Qty.	Qty. Ordered
Amoxil 500 mg	500 caps/btl	750 caps	1500 caps	_____
Lotrisone Cream	15 g/tube	3 tubes	1 tube	_____
Cephalexin 500 mg	100 caps/btl	125 caps	600 caps	_____
Ortho Novum 1/35	6 × 28 tabs/box	224 tabs	672 tabs	_____
Albuterol Inhaler	17 g/inhaler	5 inhalers	17 inhalers	_____
Robitussin AC	4 fl oz/btl	12 bottles	10 bottles	_____

Drug	Package Size	Qty on Hand	Max. Qty.	Qty. Ordered
Calan SR 240 mg	100 tabs/btl	450 tabs	625 tabs	_____
Timoptic 0.025%	15 mL/btl	2 bottles	4 bottles	_____
Fluoxetine 20 mg	30 caps/btl	12.5 bottles	19 bottles	_____
Naproxen 500 mg	100 tabs/btl	3.75 bottles	5.25 bottles	_____

Work Out the Solution

Pharm Facts—Research

Complete Table 17-1 using either the *PDR* or *Drug Facts and Comparisons.*(L-17-7)

Table 17-1

Brand Name	Generic Name	Strengths	Schedule	List One Indication of the Medication	List Three Adverse Effects of the Medication
Ambien					
Ativan					
Concerta					
Dalmane					
Darvocet N-100					
Demerol					
Dilaudid					
Hycodan					
Lunesta					
Percocet 5					
Phenobarbital					
Ritalin					
Robitussin AC					
Serax					
Stadol NS					
Tylenol with Codeine #3					
Valium					
Vicodin					
Vicodin ES					
Xanax					

Did You Know?

In 2002, the Tufts Center for the Study of Drug Development in the United States estimated the cost of drug development at $802 million. However, business consultancy, Bain and Company estimates the cost at closer to $1.7 billion. Bain and Company states that its estimate takes into consideration the costs associated with failed drug products that did not receive FDA approval. Bain and Company reported that 1 in 13 drugs makes it into preclinical development.(L-17-15)

Source: **DrugReseacher.com,** December 8, 2002.

Transition from Student to Technician

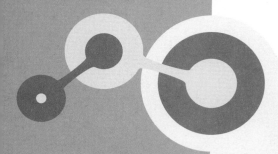

18

Preparing for Your Career as a Pharmacy Technician

Learning Outcomes

Upon completion of this laboratory chapter, you will be able to:

L-18-1 Define *externship* and explain its significance.

L-18-2 Define *professionalism*.

L-18-3 Identify expectations of the pharmacy technician student during the externship.

L-18-4 Differentiate between national certification and state board of pharmacy requirements.

L-18-5 Describe methods by which the pharmacy technician can seek employment.

L-18-6 List the components of a resume.

L-18-7 Describe pre-employment requirements.

L-18-8 List positive interviewing strategies for the job applicant.

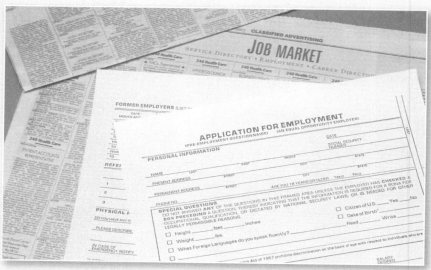

PTCB

In preparation for the certification examination, you should understand and perform activities associated with the following PTCB Knowledge Statement:

Domain III. Participating in the Administration and Management of Pharmacy Practice

> Knowledge of productivity, efficiency, and customer satisfaction (4)
>
> Knowledge of roles and responsibilities of pharmacists, pharmacy technicians, and other pharmacy employees (7)

Introduction to Preparing for Your Career(L-18-2)

As you prepare to embark on your career as a pharmacy professional, it is critical that you not only are a competent and knowledgeable pharmacy technician, but that you also possess the professional skills that will make you an excellent candidate for employment. Development of professional skills is critical to your success. The purpose of this laboratory chapter is to provide a forum in which you, the pharmacy technician student, can identify strategies and demonstrate the professional skills needed for a career as a pharmacy technician.

Test Your Knowledge

Multiple Choice Questions

Answer the following multiple choice questions. When you have finished, check your answers and then review those areas that need improvement.

1. Pharmacy technician students attend lectures and take written examinations primarily in the _____ of the pharmacy technician program.(L-18-1, 18-3)
   a. didactic courses
   b. laboratory courses
   c. externship
   d. none of the above

2. A mock pharmacy environment is often employed in the _____ courses in the pharmacy technician program.(L-18-1, 18-3)
   a. didactic
   b. laboratory
   c. experiential
   d. all of the above

3. Which of the following organizations is responsible for accreditation for pharmacy technician programs?(L-18-5)
   a. Food and Drug Administration
   b. Pharmacy Technician Certification Board
   c. American Pharmacist Association
   d. American Society of Health-System Pharmacists

4. Networking involves(L-18-6)
   a. meeting colleagues.
   b. participating in professional events.
   c. meeting potential employers.
   d. all of the above.

5. Which of the following constitutes professional behavior?(L-18-1, 18-2, 18-3)
   a. Matching wits with your instructor
   b. Arriving on time
   c. Wearing a clean, wrinkled lab coat
   d. Avoiding eye contact when talking to instructors and patients

6. Which of the following is *not* a component of the resume?(L-18-7)
   a. Contact information
   b. Employment history
   c. Education
   d. All of the above are components of the resume

7. Which of the following is *not* included in a cover letter?(L-18-6)
   a. Introduction
   b. Educational background
   c. Employment background
   d. Salary history

8. Which of the following is *not* a part of the personal portfolio?(L-18-6, 18-8)
   a. Resume
   b. Letters of recommendation
   c. Immunization records
   d. Documentation of certification

9. Which of the following should a pharmacy technician do to prepare for an interview?(L-18-9)
   a. Research the prospective employer's organization
   b. Determine responses to appropriate interview questions
   c. Draft a few questions to ask the interviewer
   d. All of the above

10. Which of the following should *not* be brought to the interview?(L-18-2, 18-9)
    a. Copies of your license/registration
    b. Additional copies of the resume
    c. Pen
    d. Chewing gum

11. Which of the following is *not* appropriate during an interview?(L-18-6, 18-8, 18-9)
    a. Maintaining eye contact
    b. Responding to questions clearly
    c. Identifying future career goals
    d. Attempting to entertain the interviewers

12. Which of the following is a good strategy to employ for a job interview?(L-18-9)
    a. Arrange for lunch for the prospective employer
    b. Arrange to have your friend accompany you to the interview
    c. Arrange to arrive at least ten minutes early
    d. None of the above

13. Which of the following is true regarding attitude?(L-18-2)
    a. It has no bearing on whether or not you are hired
    b. It does not show in your tone of voice or facial expressions
    c. It can affect your relationship with a future employer
    d. None of the above

14. Which of the following should you *not* do following an interview?(L-18-6, 18-9)
    a. Send a letter of thanks
    b. Thank the interviewer(s) for the interview
    c. Call the interviewer(s) daily until you are offered the job
    d. Offer to provide references

15. Which of the following should *not* be worn during an interview?(L-18-9)
    a. White shirt
    b. Dark suit
    c. Polished shoes
    d. Sunglasses

16. When answering questions during an interview, it is important to(L-18-2, 18-9)
    a. maintain eye contact.
    b. speak clearly and be concise.
    c. display a professional attitude.
    d. all of the above.

17. Which of the following is an appropriate question for an interviewer to ask an applicant?(L-18-9)
    a. Do you attend church on Sunday?
    b. Are you married?
    c. When would you be able to start work?
    d. Do you have young children?

18. Which of the following questions should you be able to answer in preparation for an interview?(L-18-8, 18-9)
    a. What are your greatest strengths?
    b. How do you respond to a challenge?
    c. Where do you see yourself professionally in 5 years?
    d. All of the above

19. Which of the following should you *not* do when completing an application for employment?(L-18-6, 18-8)
    a. Type or write the answers clearly
    b. Embellish your responses
    c. Indicate the items that are not applicable to you
    d. None of the above items are appropriate

20. In preparation for applying for a job, the pharmacy technician should be prepared to(L-18-4, 18-8)
    a. take a drug screening test.
    b. complete an employment application.
    c. provide proof of education/certification/registration.
    d. all of the above.

21. In addition to question 20, the pharmacy technician should be prepared to(L-18-8)
    a. take a pre-employment physical examination.
    b. provide proof of immunizations.
    c. provide proof of voter registration.
    d. a and b.

22. In the event that you are not offered the position you applied for, you should(L-18-2, 18-6)
    a. learn from the experience to determine how to improve your chances in the future.
    b. complain to your pharmacy technician instructor that the process was unfair.
    c. choose another profession.
    d. allow the experience to discourage you from applying for other positions.

23. When mailing your resume it should be accompanied by a[L-18-6]
    a. copy of your emergency contact information.
    b. copy of your Social Security card.
    c. cover letter.
    d. none of the above.

24. When faxing your resume to a prospective employer, you should include a[L-18-6]
    a. fax cover sheet.
    b. copy of your immunization records.
    c. copy of your high school diploma.
    d. all of the above.

25. N/A on a job application means[L-18-6]
    a. no answer.
    b. not applicable.
    c. never ask.
    d. not available.

Apply Your Knowledge

Read each of the actions below and determine if they are acceptable. Answer A for acceptable and U for unacceptable in the space provided.

1. _____ Sending a cover letter with a resume for an advertised position.[L-18-6]
2. _____ E-mailing your resume to a prospective employer without a cover letter or e-mail message.[L-18-2, L-18-6]
3. _____ Being asked by a prospective employer if you are certified.[L-18-4]
4. _____ Being asked by a prospective employer to take a pre-employment physical examination.[L-18-8]
5. _____ Being asked by a prospective employer about your ethnic background.[L-18-2]
6. _____ Researching the prospective employer's company on the Internet to prepare for an interview.[L-18-2, 18-9]
7. _____ Submitting an application for employment with some items left blank.[L-18-2]
8. _____ Insulting the interviewer after being told that you did not get the position for which you applied.[L-18-2]
9. _____ Practicing answering potential interview questions in a mock setting with your classmates.[L-18-9]
10. _____ Asking your pharmacy technician instructor for advice prior to going for a job interview.[L-18-1, 18-9]
11. _____ Embellishing your resume to make yourself look good to increase your chances of getting hired.[L-18-2]
12. _____ Refusing to provide information to a prospective employer regarding your religious affiliation.[L-18-2]
13. _____ Refusing to submit to a pre-employment drug test.[L-18-8]
14. _____ Interrupting the prospective employer during the interview.[L-18-2, 18-9]
15. _____ Answering your cell phone during an interview.[L-18-2, 18-9]

Practice Your Knowledge

Materials Needed

1. Paper
2. Pen
3. Computer
4. Printer
5. Newspaper advertisement
6. Internet access

Goal

To engage students in practicing the various activities associated with applying for employment.[L-18-2, 18-3, 18-6, 18-7]

Assignment

1. Prepare a resume you would present to a potential employer (typed on high-quality paper).[L-18-7]
2. Search the Internet and/or newspaper classified advertisements for available pharmacy technician positions. Choose at least two announcements for positions in different pharmacy settings.[L-18-6]
3. Draft specific cover letters for each advertisement.[L-18-6]

4. Bring copies of the announcements to present in class.[(L-18-6)]

5. Be prepared to read your cover letters to the class and discuss how the letters are different.[(L-18-6)]

6. Present your resume with cover letters to the class for review and feedback.[(L-18-2)]

Evaluation Form

Practice the task until you are able to obtain a fair or excellent self-evaluation, then obtain a final evaluation from your instructor.

Task	Self-Evaluation			Instructor Evaluation		
	Rating			Rating		
Resume Writing	Excellent	Fair	Poor	Excellent	Fair	Poor
Resume presents a professional image						
Resume is free of typographical and grammatical errors						
Resume is organized to highlight your best characteristics						
Resume is factual						
Cover letters are appropriate for the positions for which you are "applying"						
Cover letters are free of grammatical and typographical errors						
Cover letters provide the prospective employer with the impression that you are interested in the position, and that you possess the qualities and traits necessary for the position						

Which letter do you prefer and why?[(L-18-2)]
Which letter do your classmates prefer?[(L-18-2)]
What feedback have they provided?[(L-18-2)]

Based upon your self-assessment and that of your instructor and classmates, would you modify your letter after this exercise? Why or why not?[(L-18-6, 18-8)]

Calculation Corner

The BestRx Pharmacy has offered you a job at $32,000 annually for full-time employment with fringe benefits calculated at 29%. Calculate your salary adjusted to include fringe benefits.[(L-18-8)]

Work Out the Solution

Did You Know

According to the U.S. Department of Labor Statistics Occupational Outlook, 2008–2009, employment for the pharmacy technicians is expected to increase much faster than the average through 2016, and job opportunities are expected to be good.

Career Development

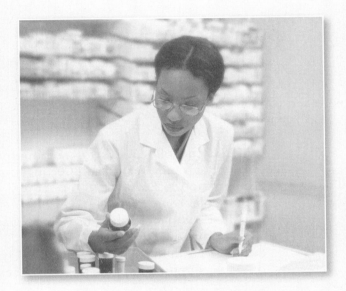

19

Learning Outcomes

Upon completion of this laboratory chapter, you will be able to:

L-19-1 Identify stress management strategies.

L-19-2 Identify time management strategies.

L-19-3 Describe the role of the employee evaluation in career development.

L-19-4 Differentiate between certification and registration.

L-19-5 Describe the role of continuing education in the maintenance of professional status.

L-19-6 List pharmacy organizations and describe their purposes.

PTCB

In preparation for the certification examination, you should understand and perform activities associated with the following PTCB Knowledge Statement:

Domain III. Participating in the Administration and Management of Pharmacy Practice

Knowledge of required operational licenses and certificates (6)

Knowledge of employee performance evaluation (37)

Introduction to Career Development(L-19-1, 19-5, 19-6)

It is important to get a good start on your career as a pharmacy technician. All of the concepts, skills, and techniques you acquired in the pharmacy technician program now must be put into action. This laboratory chapter reviews the various aspects of career development including handling on-the-job issues, maintaining registration and certification, and becoming involved in professional organizations.

Test Your Knowledge

Multiple Choice Questions

Answer the following multiple choice questions. When you have finished, check your answers and then review those areas that need improvement.

1. Which of the following organizations is responsible for certification of pharmacy technicians?(L-19-4, 19-6)
   a. AAPT
   b. ASHP
   c. PTCB
   d. PTEC

2. Which of the following organizations is responsible for registration or licensure of pharmacy technicians?(L-19-4, 19-6)
   a. Food and Drug Administration
   b. State Board of Pharmacy
   c. Centers for Disease Control and Prevention
   d. National Pharmacy Technician Association

3. Which of the following organizations is responsible for accreditation of pharmacy technician programs?(L-19-6)
   a. NABP
   b. AAPT
   c. ASHP
   d. NPTA

4. Which of the following organizations was established for pharmacy technicians educators?(L-19-6)
   a. PTCB
   b. ASHP
   c. PTEC
   d. AAPT

5. Which of the following is *not* a requirement for the Pharmacy Technician Certification Examination?(L-19-4)
   a. Must be 18 years of age
   b. Must complete a pharmacy technician program
   c. Must pay a fee for the exam
   d. Must submit an application for the exam

6. CPhT means(L-19-4)
   a. certified pharmacy trainee.
   b. certified pharmacy technician.
   c. certified pharmaceutical trainee.
   d. certified pharmacist trainee.

7. Which of the following is *not* a requirement for renewal of the CPhT?(L-19-5)
   a. Must have twenty hours of continuing education over 2 years.
   b. A component of the continuing education must be in pharmacy law.
   c. A fee must be paid.
   d. The exam must be taken again.

8. Which of the following is *not* a certifying agency for pharmacy technicians?(L-19-4, 19-6)
   a. NCCT
   b. PTCB
   c. ICPT
   d. AAPT

9. Which of the following organizations was founded specifically for pharmacy technicians?(L-19-6)
   a. NCCT
   b. NPTA
   c. APhA
   d. ASHP

10. Which of the following organizations accredits/approves continuing education providers?(L-19-5, 19-6)
    a. ASHP
    b. ACPE
    c. AAPT
    d. APhA

11. Which of the following is *not* an appropriate stress management technique?(L-19-1)
    a. Resist the urge to take on too much too soon; you cannot do everything.
    b. Arrive on time and be ready to work.
    c. Skip your breaks and lunch periods.
    d. Know when to ask for help.

12. Which of the following is not an appropriate time management technique?(L-19-2)
    a. Be on time.
    b. Try to do everything at once.
    c. Start a task and follow it through to completion.
    d. Plan how you use your time.

13. Another term for employee evaluation form is(L-19-3)
    a. certification form.
    b. performance appraisal form.
    c. verification form.
    d. none of the above.

14. Which of the following criteria for evaluation is *not* likely to appear on a pharmacy technician' performance appraisal form?(L-19-3)
    a. Competence
    b. Safety
    c. Initiative
    d. Intelligence

15. One hour of continuing education credit is identified as(L-19-5)
    a. 0.01 CEU.
    b. 0.1 CEU.
    c. 1 CEU.
    d. 10 CEU.

16. _____ accredits continuing education providers.(L-19-5, 19-6)
    a. ACPE
    b. TJC, formerly JCAHO
    c. ASHP
    d. PTCB

17. Which of the following is a benefit of participation in professional organizations?(L-19-6)
    a. Employment opportunities
    b. Networking
    c. Opportunities for advocacy for the profession
    d. All of the above

18. Which of the following is false regarding employee evaluations?(L-19-3)
    a. The review is recorded in writing.
    b. The employee's work performance is the primary criteria for evaluation.
    c. The employee's personality is the primary criteria for evaluation.
    d. The employee must sign the completed form.

19. How many CEUs of pharmacy law continuing education are needed to maintain PTCB certification?(L-19-4, 19-5)
    a. 0.1
    b. 1
    c. 10
    d. 20

20. Which of the following is a benefit of professional organizations?(L-19-6)
    a. Recognition among peers
    b. Opportunities for scholarships and awards
    c. Leadership opportunities
    d. All of the above

Matching

Match the organization's acronym with its role in pharmacy. (L-19-6)

_____ 1. PTCB

_____ 2. NPTA

_____ 3. FDA

_____ 4. ACPE

_____ 5. ASHP

A. Professional organization for pharmacy technicians

B. Regulatory agency

C. Technician program accreditation agency

D. Certifying agency

E. Continuing education approval agency

True/False

Mark True or False for each statement. If it is false, correct the statement to make it true.

1. _____ The American Pharmacists Association (APhA) was founded in 1852 and is dedicated to advancing the profession of pharmacy.(L-19-6)

2. _____ ASHP is the accrediting agency for pharmacy technician programs and for pharmacy residency programs.(L-19-6)

3. _____ The focus of NPTA is primarily the practice of pharmacists.(L-19-6)

4. _____ The Pharmacy Technician Educators Council consists primarily of pharmacy technician teachers.(L-19-6)

5. _____ The Pharmacy Technician Certification Board (PTCB) is an agency that reports to each state's board of pharmacy.(L-19-4, 19-6)

6. _____ ASHP holds several meetings annually.(L-19-6)

7. _____ Pharmacy technician participation in professional organizations helps keep the technician current with the profession.(L-19-6)

8. _____ The pharmacy technician's certificate or registration card must be kept under lock and key.(L-19-4)

9. _____ It is important for the pharmacy technician to know the requirements in his or her own state.(L-19-4)

10. _____ Some boards of pharmacy offer continuing education for attending a board meeting.(L-19-4, 19-5)

Apply Your Knowledge

1. List five stress management strategies. Why is the utilization of stress management techniques critical in the pharmacy technician's practice?(L-19-1)

_____

_____

2. List five time management strategies. How many other time management strategies (that were not discussed in the chapter)

can you list? Why is time management so important for pharmacy technicians?(L-19-2)

_____

_____

3. Identify three phases of employee evaluation. What criteria are included in employee evaluation for pharmacy technicians?(L-19-3)

_____

_____

4. Discuss the differences between registration and certification. Does your state recognize pharmacy technicians as paraprofessionals? What are the requirements in your state for practice as a pharmacy technician?(L-19-4, 19-5)

_____

_____

5. List four professional organizations while identifying the purpose for each one. What are some benefits of membership?(L-19-6)

_____

_____

Practice Your Knowledge

Materials Needed

1. Internet access
2. Telephone
3. Paper
4. Pen or pencil

Goal

To develop an understanding of the roles of pharmacy organizations as they pertain to the pharmacy technician and to engage the technician student in a local meeting to foster an appreciation for membership.(L-19-6)

Assignment

1. Identify a local professional pharmacy organization, either through searching the Internet or through discussions with your pharmacy technician instructor.(L-19-6)
2. Contact the organization, either through telephone or e-mail, to inquire about the organization's scheduled meetings.(L-19-6)
3. Attend the meeting.(L-19-6)

4. While in attendance, obtain any minutes, agendas, and announcements. (L-19-6)
5. After the meeting, return to class prepared to present the following information to the class for discussion:(L-19-5, 19-6)

   a. The name of the organization.
   b. The mission of the organization.
   c. Organization affiliation.
   d. List of officers.
   e. Frequency of meetings.
   f. Agenda items discussed at the meeting.
   g. Length of the meeting.
   h. Whether the organization offers continuing education hours for pharmacists and/or technicians. If so, in what format (face-to-face meetings, Web-based, mail-in examinations, etc.)?

6. Be prepared to discuss whether you thought the issues and concerns of pharmacy technicians were discussed in the meeting. Also, indicate whether or not you might be interested in becoming a member of the organization and provide your reasons why or why not.(L-19-6)

Calculation Corner

Assume that you have attended a few continuing education workshops and have received certificates for the following:(L-19-5)

Topic	CEU
Over-the-Counter Cough Preparations	0.2
Compounding Agents for Topical Application	0.3
Legal Updates in Pharmacy Practice	0.1
The Use of Technology in Pharmacies Serving Rural Populations	0.2

1. Knowing that 0.1 continuing education units (CEUs) is equivalent to one hour of credit, how many hours of credit have you earned? _____

2. How many more hours do you need to meet the continuing education requirements to renew certification? _____

Work Out the Solution

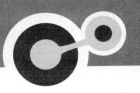

Answer Key

Chapter 1 Lab

Multiple Choice Answers

1. d—All of the above are roles of a pharmacist
   A pharmacist performs both technical and judgmental duties in the practice of pharmacy. Pharmacy practice involves both the preparation and distribution of medication and the dissemination of information to the patient and other health care providers. When pharmacists collect information from patients, they are performing a technical task. Meanwhile, counseling and providing information is a judgmental duty.
2. d—All of the above
   It is the responsibility of the pharmacist to ensure that all prescriptions are processed correctly by pharmacy technicians, Drug Utilization Evaluations are performed on all prescription and medication orders, and that medication distribution is handled properly in all settings.
3. a—Assist the pharmacist
   The pharmacy technician's primary responsibility is to assist the pharmacist. This is accomplished by performing technical duties in the pharmacy.
4. b—Technical
   Pharmacy technicians perform technical tasks in a pharmacy.
5. c—State board of pharmacy
   The state board of pharmacy is responsible for the practice of pharmacy within that state, which includes both pharmacists and pharmacy technicians.
6. d—All of the above
7. d—State board of pharmacy
   The state board of pharmacy is responsible for the practice of pharmacy in the state.
8. b—Pharmacist
   The pharmacist on duty is responsible for any work that a pharmacy technician performs during the shift.
9. d—Irresponsible
   Pharmacy technicians are responsible, not irresponsible, individuals.
10. d—All of the above
    All of the characteristics are needed for a pharmacy technician to be successful in the practice of pharmacy.

11. d—All of the above
    These are some of the many skills that a pharmacy technician should possess regardless of the pharmacy setting.
12. d—All of the above
    These are some of the many pharmacy knowledge skills that a pharmacy technician will need in the practice of pharmacy.
13. d—All of the above
    All of the tasks mentioned are technical tasks that a pharmacy technician can perform.
14. d—All of the above
    An institutional setting is a hospital setting. Aseptic technique is required in a hospital pharmacy preparing IVs. Hospital pharmacies utilize automation and robotics more than a retail pharmacy.
15. d—All of the above
    A pharmacy technician working in a facility preparing medications for long-term care patients must have a strong knowledge for repackaging medications and the processes involved. Federal law requires that a patient's medication be packaged in a unit-dose form.

True/False Answers

1. False. Pharmacy technicians need a strong basic math background, especially with the use of proportions.
2. False. Externships occur upon completion of a pharmacy technician program. An internship occurs while a pharmacy technician is in a pharmacy technician program.
3. True.
4. False. Communication is extremely important in the practice of pharmacy but pharmacy technicians are not permitted to counsel patients at this time.
5. True.
6. False. There are more retail pharmacies in the United States than hospital pharmacies.
7. True.
8. False. Approximately 30 state boards of pharmacy require either certification or registration of pharmacy technicians.

9. True.
10. False. IVs are prepared in hospital pharmacies.

Apply Your Knowledge Answers

1. Answers will vary, but should include the following: the increased number of individuals who are part of the aging population; the fact that individuals are living longer; the increased number of prescriptions being filled; the day's supply limitation due to managed care; the shortage of pharmacists.
2. Answers will vary.
3. Answers will vary.
4. Certification is the process by which an agency grants recognition to an individual who has met predetermined qualifications specified by the agency or organization. Licensure is the process by which an agency or association grants permission to an individual to engage in a particular occupation based on finding that the individual has attained a minimal degree of competency necessary to ensure that the public health, safety, and welfare will be reasonably protected.
5. Certification is being required by many employers and by the various state boards of pharmacy.
6. Assisting the pharmacist.

7. It is a requirement to remain certified, but more importantly it is necessary for a pharmacy technician to remain knowledgeable of the changes in pharmacy practice due to new medications being introduced, changes in drug therapies, and changes in pharmacy laws, to name a few.
8. Ask the physician's office to wait while you get the pharmacist to take the prescription order.
9. Answers will vary.
10. Inform the patient that you will get the pharmacist to answer his question. This is an example of counseling. Pharmacy technicians are not permitted to counsel patients.

Calculation Corner Answers

Solution

1. How many days will the prescription last?

$$\text{Day's supply} = \frac{\text{Total number of capsules dispensed}}{\text{Total number of capsules taken each day}}$$

$$\frac{40 \text{ capsules}}{4 \text{ capsules per day}} = 10 \text{ days' supply of medicine}$$

The prescription will last 10 days.

Pharmacy Facts—Research Answers

Table 1-1

Brand Name	Generic Name	Strengths	Dosage Forms	List One Indication of the Medication	List Five Adverse Effects of the Medication
Achromycin	tetracycline	250 and 500 mg	Capsule	Bacterial infection	Answers will vary
Amoxil	amoxicillin	500 mg 200 mg/5 mL 250 mg/5 mL 400 mg/5 mL 500 mg 875 mg 400 mg	Capsule Suspension Tablet Chewable tablet	Bacterial infection	Answers will vary
Augmentin	amoxicillin + clauvanate	250/125 mg 500/125 mg 875/125 mg 125/31 mg 250/62.5 mg 400/57 mg 250/62.5 mg 400/57.5 mg	Tablet Chewable tablets Suspension	Bacterial infection	Answers will vary
Bactrim DS	trimethoprim/ sulfamethoxazole	160/800 mg	Tablet	Bacterial infection	Answers will vary
Biaxin	clarithromycin	250 and 500 mg 125 mg/5 mL 250 mg/5 mL	Tablet Suspension	Bacterial infection	Answers will vary
Ceclor	cefaclor	250 mg 500 mg 375 mg 500 mg	Capsule Extended release tablet	Bacterial infection	Answers will vary

(Continued)

Table 1-1   *(Continued)*

Brand Name	Generic Name	Strengths	Dosage Forms	List One Indication of the Medication	List Five Adverse Effects of the Medication
Ceftin	Cefuroxime	250 mg 500 mg	Tablet	Bacterial infection	Answers will vary
Cipro	Ciprofloxacin	100 mg 250 mg 500 mg 750 mg 250 mg/5 mL 500 mg/5 mL 400 mg	Tablet Suspension IV	Bacterial infection	Answers will vary
Cleocin	clindamycin	75 mg 150 mg 300 mg 75 mg/5 mL	Capsule Suspension	Bacterial infection	Answers will vary
Duracef	cefadroxil	500 mg 1 g 250 mg 500 mg	Capsule Tablet Suspension	Bacterial infection	Answers will vary
E.E.S.	erythromycin ethyl succinate	200 mg 400 mg 400 mg	Suspension Film tab Granules	Bacterial infection	Answers will vary
Flagyl	metronidazole	250 mg 500 mg	Tablets	Bacterial infection	Answers will vary
Floxin	ofloxacin	200 mg 400 mg	Tablets	Bacterial infection	Answers will vary
Gantrisin	sulfisoxazole	500 mg/5 mL	Suspension	Bacterial infection	Answers will vary
Garamycin	gentamicin	0.3 %	Suspension	Bacterial infection	Answers will vary
Keflex	cephalexin	250 mg 333 mg 500 mg 750 mg	Capsule	Bacterial infection	Answers will vary
Lorabid	loracarbef	200 mg 400 mg	Pulvules	Bacterial infection	Answers will vary
Macrodantin	nitrofurantoin	25 mg 50 mg 100 mg	Capsules	Urinary tract infection	Answers will vary
Minocin	minocycline	50 mg 100 mg	Capsule	Acne	Answers will vary
Pen Vee K	penicillin vk	250 mg 500 mg 125 mg/5 mL 250 mg/5 mL	Tablet Suspension	Bacterial infection	Answers will vary
Rocephin	ceftriaxone	500 mg 1 g	Vial	Bacterial infection	Answers will vary
Vancocin	vancomycin	125 mg 250 mg	Capsule	Bacterial infection	Answers will vary
Vantin	cefpodoxime	100 mg 200 mg	Tablet	Bacterial infection	Answers will vary
Vibramycin	doxycycline	100 mg 25 mg 50 mg/5 mL	Capsule Suspension Syrup	Bacterial infection	Answers will vary
Zithromax	azithromycin	250 mg 500 mg 600 mg 100 mg/5 mL 200 mg/5 mL 1 g	Tablet Suspension Packet	Bacterial infection	Answers will vary

Chapter 2 Lab
Multiple Choice Answers

1. a—An infection acquired in an inpatient setting
Nosocomial refers to a specific category of infections that occur in inpatient or institutionalized settings as a result of poor infection control.

2. c—Multiple-drug resistance
Infections that are not managed with more than one antimicrobial agent may be due to bacteria that have developed multiple-drug resistance.

3. c—Human papillomavirus
Hepatitis B, HIV, and hepatitis C are all transmitted via the bloodstream. The human papillomavirus is transmitted via touch or direct contact.

4. b—Saliva
Cerebrospinal fluid, semen, and synovial fluid are all considered infectious, regardless of whether they contain blood. Saliva is considered infectious only if it contains blood.

5. c—Two, 4
The CDC recommends treatment with at least two antiretroviral agents for at least 4 weeks after an occupational exposure to HIV.

6. a—A prophylactic regimen should begin within hours of exposure
The CDC recommends that the prophylactic regimen begin within hours of exposure.

7. d—All patients
Standard precautions should be followed in all health care settings.

8. b—The size of the particles transmitted
The main difference in droplet transmission and airborne transmission of pathogens is the size of the particles. Airborne transmission involves the transmission of droplet particles less than 5 micrometers in size, while droplet transmission involves droplet particles greater than 5 micrometers.

9. b—Holding his or her breath while in the same room with a patient
Employing proper hand hygiene and proper use of protective wear helps prevent contact transmission. Holding one's breath will not prevent contact transmission.

10. c—Gloveless hand shake
Hand washing and the proper use of antiseptics on the hands are components of hand hygiene. Shaking hands or touching without gloves is not a component of hand hygiene.

11. d—Multidrug-resistant pathogens
Multidrug-resistant pathogens are impervious or resistant to more than one antibacterial agent.

12. b—Maintain product sterility
Aseptic technique is used to maintain product sterility.

13. b—CDC
The Centers for Disease Control and Prevention (CDC) is primarily concerned with the control and prevention of disease.

14. c—OSHA
The Occupational Safety and Health Administration (OSHA) is primarily concerned with workplace safety.

15. c—Smallpox
Smallpox is not a food borne disease. Salmonella, shigella, and botulism are all food borne pathogens.

16. a—EAP
The Emergency Action Plan (EAP) is a document that is designed to facilitate and organize actions in the event of a workplace emergency.

17. b—FPP
The Fire Prevention Plan (FPP) consists of a list of potential workplace fire hazards and types and locations of fire control devices.

18. d—Triclosan
Ricin, smallpox, and anthrax are pathogens that have been associated with bioterrorism. Triclosan is an antiseptic agent to prevent pathogen transmission.

19. b—Using appropriate personal protective equipment
Appropriately using personal protective equipment does not contribute to pharmacy technician exposure to hazardous substances.

20. d—Horizontal biologic safety cabinet
A horizontal biologic safety cabinet is not appropriate for the preparation of hazardous substances as it increases the risk of drug exposure.

21. c—Wearing two pairs of gloves while working in the BSC
Wearing two pairs of gloves while working in the BSC *reduces* the risk of exposure.

22. a—Storage of nonsterile products
The Joint Commission has recommendations regarding the storage of sterile products but not nonsterile products in the Pharmacy Infection Control Policies and Procedures.

23. b—Zovirax (acyclovir)
Zovirax is not a component of HIV post exposure prophylaxis; it is an antiviral commonly prescribed to treat infections caused by the herpes virus.

24. b—EPA
The Environmental Protection Agency (EPA) provides standards for hazardous waste disposal.

True/False Answers

1. False. The use of gloves does not eliminate the need for hand washing.
2. False. Nosocomial infections are contracted within the health care setting.
3. True.
4. True.

5. False. Synovial fluid is considered potentially infectious regardless of whether it contains blood.
6. True.
7. True.
8. True.
9. False. The pharmacy technician is responsible for assisting the pharmacist in controlling and preventing infection in the pharmacy.
10. False. According to OSHA standards, employers must retain an Emergency Action Plan (EAP) and a Fire Prevention Plan (FPP).
11. True.

Apply Your Knowledge Answers

1. Answers will vary, but should include the following: anthrax, Avian flu, hepatitis B, hepatitis C, HIV, salmonella, shigella, hantavirus, Legionnaires' disease, ricin, plague, botulism, severe acute respiratory syndrome, smallpox, tularemia, viral hemorrhagic fever.
2. The incident report is used for internal reporting. External reports to the CDC, police departments, fire departments, and local health departments are required in the event of outbreaks of infectious disease, for example. Suspected bioterrorist attacks should also be reported to the FBI.
3. Carcinogenicity, teratogenicity, reproductive toxicity, organ toxicity at low doses, and genotoxicity
4. Answers will vary, but should include the following:
   - Access to area where hazardous materials are stored should be restricted.
   - Hazardous materials should be separated from nonhazardous agents, even in the refrigerator.
   - Solid plastic bins should be used to decrease leakage in case of breakage.
   - Food and/or beverages should never be stored in the same area or refrigerator with any drug products.
   - Warning labels should be applied to all bins containing hazardous materials.
5. Answers will vary, but should include the following: asparaginase, azathioprine, bicalutamide, bleomycin, carmustine, chloramphenicol, dacarbazine, estradiol, fluoxymesterone, lomustine, mifepristone, mitomycin, nafarelin, oxytocin, progesterone, raloxifene, ribavirin, tacrolimus, thioguanine, tretinonin, vidarabine, vincristine, zidovudine.

Calculation Corner Answers

Solution

1. How many milliliters will be required for each dose?

   150 mg/X mL = 125 mg/5 mL
   X = 150 mg × 5 mL/125 mg

X = 6 mL
6 mL will be required for each dose.

2. What is the minimum amount of amoxicillin needed for the prescription? There are 150 mg in 6 mL. One dose every 8 hours equals 3 doses daily for 10 days:

   6 mL × 3 doses/day × 10 days = 180 mL
   X = 180 mL

   180 mL is the minimum amount of amoxicillin needed for the prescription.

Chapter 3 Lab
Multiple Choice Answers

1. d —All of the above
   Communication can be either upward, downward, or lateral.
2. c—The height of the pharmacy counter
   The height of the pharmacy counter can act as a barrier between the patient and the pharmacy staff in the communication process. The counter height can prevent the patient and the pharmacy staff from hearing correctly what the other individual is saying.
3. d—All of the above
   Looking, smiling, and speaking to the customer are all examples of positive communication.
4. d—All of the above
   Asking questions, listening for the individual to express his or her feelings, and paraphrasing what an individual is saying are examples of active listening.
5. c—Interrupting the patient
   Interrupting the patient is not an example of good telephone etiquette. It demonstrates to the patient that you are not actively listening.
6. b—Factors affecting the ability to speak and understand English
   The ability to speak and understand English does not affect the ability to interpret nonverbal communication.
7. a—Kinesics
   Kinesics is a form of nonverbal communication that involves body movement and facial expressions. Oculesics involves the use of colors to communicate to individuals. Proxemics uses distance between individuals as a method of communication.
8. b—Personal
   Personal distance is used in collecting information from a patient.
9. d—All of the above
   A customer may become angry with the pharmacy staff when a prescription error occurs. He or she

may develop anxiety wondering how the wrong medication has affected him or her. The customer may be confused about how and why the prescription error occurred.

10. d—Resentment

There are five stages a terminally ill patient may experience: denial, anger, bargaining, depression, and acceptance. Resentment is not one of the stages.

11. d—All of the above

An individual may experience emotional, mental, and physical problems from continual stress. These problems will vary from individual to individual.

12. a—Human resource department of your employer

The human resource department of an employer is an internal customer, not an external customer. A nurse, patient, or physician would be considered an external customer of the pharmacy.

13. a—ACPE

The Accreditation Council for Pharmacy Education (ACPE) is responsible for accrediting all continuing education for pharmacy technicians.

14. d—70%

Pharmacy technicians must receive a minimum score of 70% to receive credit for continuing education courses.

15. d—All of the above

Shyness may be a social or psychological barrier, the height of the counter may be a physical barrier, and time may be a cultural barrier in the communication process.

True/False Answers

1. True.
2. True.
3. True.
4. False. Listening is an active process.
5. True.
6. False. Empathy is being able to communicate to an individual that you are able to understand his or her feelings in a caring manner. Sympathy exists when the feelings of one person are deeply understood and appreciated by another person.
7. True.
8. True.
9. True.
10. True.
11. True.
12. True.
13. True.
14. True.
15. True.

Matching Answers

1. F	3. B	5. C	7. J	9. A
2. I	4. H	6. G	8. E	10. D

Apply Your Knowledge Answers

1.
   a. There are no remaining refills on the prescription and the pharmacy is unable to contact the physician for permission to refill the prescription.
   b. Ask the patient if she is completely out of the medication. If she is, ask the pharmacist if you can provide her with enough of the medication to last until you can obtain permission from the physician on Monday.

2.
   a. Yes. Mr. Kunze provided the pharmacy with all of the necessary prescription and personal information to refill the prescription.
   b. A member of the pharmacy staff should have notified Mr. Kunze as soon as possible that they were experiencing problems obtaining refill permission from his physician. The pharmacy should have made multiple attempts to contact Mr. Kunze's physician.
   c. Apologize to the patient. Call the physician's office immediately for refill authorization. If you are unable to obtain refill authorization, ask the pharmacist if you may provide the patient with enough medication until the patient can return to pick up the medication.
   d. The problem could have been avoided if someone from the pharmacy had been persistent in contacting the physician's office and notifying the patient of any problems encountered.

3.
   a. The pharmacy technician could offer to order the medication for the patient to be delivered on its next scheduled delivery from a wholesaler, or could attempt to locate the medication at another pharmacy for the patient.
   b. Explain politely to Mr. Dagit the situation and the possible alternatives and ask him how he would like the pharmacy to proceed.
   c. The technician handled the situation properly by promptly asking the pharmacist the in-stock status of the medication.

4. A clean, neat, organized, and well-lit pharmacy will convey to the customer the attention to detail the pharmacy staff demonstrates. However, a dirty, sloppy, and poorly lit pharmacy may give the customer the opposite impression.

5. If someone accompanied Ms. Vargas to the pharmacy, the technician could ask her friend for the necessary information. Another possibility would be if someone in the pharmacy spoke the same language as Ms. Vargas.

6. The answers will vary based on the student's personal experiences.

7. The answers will vary but possible habits might include punctuality, attention to detail, strong

communications skills, and ability to work with a variety of people.

8. A pharmacy technician is considered a paraprofessional because his or her primary responsibility is to assist the pharmacist.
9. Listen carefully and demonstrate empathy toward the patient.
10. Demonstrations will vary depending on the medication dispensed.

Practice Your Knowledge Answers

The student's observation will vary based on the pharmacy and the situations he or she observed. The exercise will allow the student to see a situation through a customer's eyes.

The students should participate actively in this exercise. Each group of two students should take turns role playing the technician and the patient.

Pharmacy Facts—Research Answers

Table 3-1

Brand Name	Generic Name	Strengths	Indications	Contraindication	Adverse Effect
Anusol HC Suppositories	hydrocortisone	25 mg	hemorrhoids	Answers will vary	Answers will vary
Bactrim Pediatric Suspension	sulfamethoixazole/ trimethoprim	200 mg/40 mg per teaspoon	infections (ear and urinary tract)	Answers will vary	Answers will vary
Cortisporin TC Otic Suspension	colistin sulfate/ neomycin sulfate/ thonzonium bromide/ hydrocortisone acetate	This medication does not come in multiple strengths	ear infections	Answers will vary	Answers will vary
Domeboro Tablets	aluminum acetate	1:40	topical astringent	Answers will vary	Answers will vary
EES Chewable Tablets	erythromycin	200 mg	bacterial infections	Answers will vary	Answers will vary
Epi-Pen	epinephrine	0.3 mg	anaphylactic reactions	Answers will vary	Answers will vary
Epsom Salts	magnesium sulfate	Does not have a strength	topical soaks and laxative	Answers will vary	Answers will vary
Fleet Enema	sodium biphosphate and sodium phosphate	Does not have a strength	laxative	Answers will vary	Answers will vary
Flonase	fluticasone	50 mcg/spray	respiratory allergy	Answers will vary	Answers will vary
Humulin 70/30 Insulin	human insulin isophane suspension and human insulin injection	70% human insulin isophane suspension and 30% human insulin injection (rDNA origin)	insulin-dependent diabetes mellitus	Answers will vary	Answers will vary

Calculation Corner Answers

Solution

1. How many milliliters would the patient need to draw up in the syringe with each injection? The problem can be solved by using a proportion:

100 units/1 mL = 35 units/X mL

Cross-multiply:

(100 units)(X mL) = (1 mL) (35 units)

Divide both sides of the equation by 100 units:

$$\frac{(100 \text{ units}) (X \text{ mL})}{100 \text{ units}} = \frac{(1 \text{ mL}) (35 \text{ units})}{100 \text{ units}}$$

$$X = 0.35 \text{ mL}$$

The patient would need to draw up 0.35 mL of insulin with each injection.

(Continued)

Table 3-1   *(Continued)*

Brand Name	Generic Name	Strengths	Indications	Contraindication	Adverse Effect
Keflex Capsules	cephalexin	250 mg, 333 mg, 500 mg and 750 mg	bacterial infections	Answers will vary	Answers will vary
Lotrimin Cream	clotrimazole	1%	fungal infections	Answers will vary	Answers will vary
Metamucil	psyllium	Does not have a strength	laxative	Answers will vary	Answers will vary
Monistat 7 Vaginal Cream	miconazole	2%	fungal infections	Answers will vary	Answers will vary
Mycelex Troche	clotrimazole	10 mg	fungal infections	Answers will vary	Answers will vary
Nitrostat	nitroglycerin	0.3 mg (1/200 gr), 0.4 mg (1/150 gr), 0.6 mg (1/100 gr)	angina	Answers will vary	Answers will vary
Nizoral Shampoo	ketoconazole	1%	topical fungal infections	Answers will vary	Answers will vary
Ocean Nasal Spray	normal saline solution	0.9%	nasal decongestant	Answers will vary	Answers will vary
St. Joseph's Chewable Aspirin	acetylsalicylic acid	81 mg	analgesic, antipyretic and anti-inflammatory	Answers will vary	Answers will vary
Tessalon Perles	benzonatate	100 mg	cough suppressant	Answers will vary	Answers will vary
Timoptic Ophthalmic Drops	timolol	0.25%, 0.5%	glaucoma	Answers will vary	Answers will vary
Tylenol Pediatric Drops	acetaminophen	80 mg/5 mL	analgesic and antipyretic	Answers will vary	Answers will vary
Zovirax Ointment	acyclovir	5%	viral infections	Answers will vary	Answers will vary

Chapter 4 Lab

Multiple Choice Answers

1. c—Manufacturer, drug, and package size
   An NDC number consists of three components that identify the drug manufacturer, the drug entity, and the drug's packaging.
2. b—Established conditions for drugs that should not be in a child-resistant container
   The Poison Prevention Act of 1970 established specific conditions that allow for a medication to be dispensed in non-child-resistant packaging. Some of these conditions include a request by the prescriber or the patient and specific medications.
3. a—Mandated Drug Utilization Evaluation
   One of the conditions of OBRA-90 mandated that a Drug Utilization Evaluation be performed on every medication that is prescribed for a patient.
4. a—The development of generic drugs and new drug products
   The Drug Price Competition and Patent Term Restoration Act of 1984 outlined the process for the development of new drug entities and the approval process for generic medications after a medication's patent had expired.
5. d—All of the above are exemptions
6. d—All of the above
   Sublingual nitroglycerin tablets, oral contraceptives, and inhalation aerosols are a few of the

medications that do not need to be packaged in a child-resistant container.

7. b—To develop pharmaceutical products with a limited use by providing manufacturers tax incentives and exclusive licenses

The Orphan Drug Act of 1983 provided tax incentives to drug manufacturers and exclusive licensing for specific medications where there are less than 200,000 cases in the world. Without this legislation, drug manufacturers may not allocate the appropriate resources for drug research for specific conditions.

8. d—All of the above

The Prescription Drug Marketing Act of 1987 was enacted to eliminate secondary distribution markets for medications. This was accomplished by preventing the reimportation of drugs into the United States other than by the drug manufacturer, and by prohibiting the sale or trading of drug samples and barring the distribution of samples other than to individuals who are licensed to prescribe them.

9. e—a and b only

OBRA-90 required that a Drug Utilization Evaluation (Review) be conducted on every prescription or medication order dispensed by a pharmacy. Also, an offer must be made to counsel each patient regarding his or her medication.

10. d—All of the above

Drug Utilization Evaluation (Review) includes the screening of potential drug therapy problems due to therapeutic duplication, and evaluating drug-disease contraindications and drug-drug interactions.

11. d—All of the above

Under OBRA-90, counseling can take many forms whether it is done verbally or through the dissemination of print materials. Counseling could include providing the patient the name of the medication prescribed; communicating any special directions involving the preparation, storage, or use of the medication by the patient; or by informing the patient of possible side effects he or she may experience while taking the medication.

12. c—Loss of Medicaid participation

A pharmacy may be prevented from participating in Medicaid if it fails to adhere to OBRA-90.

13. d—Refilled prescriptions may be called in to the pharmacy

Legislation was enacted to prevent the teratogenic effects of Accutane. This legislation outlined what conditions must be met when prescribing Accutane and filling an Accutane prescription. Although Accutane is not a controlled substance, it requires a handwritten prescription and cannot be called in to a pharmacy by a physician's office.

14. d—Men must undergo a pregnancy test

Men do not need to take a pregnancy test to have an Accutane prescription filled.

15. b—To provide comprehensive privacy for all patients in the United States

HIPAA was passed to provide comprehensive privacy for all patients regardless of the health care setting.

16. a—FDA

The Food and Drug Administration (FDA) is responsible for the purity, safety, and efficacy of all medications on the market in the United States.

17. b—DEA

The Drug Enforcement Administration (DEA), under the Department of Justice, places a medication within a particular schedule. This decision is dependent on whether a medication has an approved medical use and whether it possesses either physical or psychological dependency.

18. d—State boards of pharmacy

Each state has its own board of pharmacy that oversees the practice of pharmacy within the state. The board of pharmacy oversees pharmacies, pharmacists, and pharmacy technicians.

19. c—TJC

The Joint Commission (TJC), formerly known as The Joint Commission on the Accreditation of Healthcare Organizations (JCAHO), is responsible for accrediting hospitals, home health care agencies, and long-term care facilities. Failure to receive this accreditation prevents an institution from receiving Medicare funds.

20. d—DSHEA 1994

The Dietary Supplement Health and Education Act prevents a manufacturer from making a disease claim.

21. c—Prescription Drug Marketing Act of 1987

The Prescription Drug Marketing Act of 1987 prohibited the sale or distribution of pharmaceutical samples to anyone other than those licensed to prescribe them. This legislation prevented drug salespeople from providing samples to pharmacies.

22. a—Federal law prohibits dispensing without a prescription

The federal legend has since been replaced with "Rx Only."

23. d—WO1234563

The first letter of a DEA number is either an "A," "B," "F," or "M." In this example the first letter is a "W" which indicates that it is not a valid number.

24. d—To prohibit the interstate transportation or sale of adulterated and misbranded food and drugs

The Pure Food and Drug Act of 1906 was passed to prohibit the interstate transportation or sale of adulterated or misbranded food and drugs.

25. c—To ensure that all food and drugs were pure, safe, and effective

The Kefauver-Harris Amendment of the Food, Drug and Cosmetic Act of 1938 ensures that all food and drugs are pure, safe, and effective for use.

26. c—Physician's supervision
An individual does not need a physician's supervision to purchase an over-the-counter (OTC) medication.

27. b—DEA Form 106
A DEA Form 106 is used to document a theft of controlled substances from a pharmacy.

28. c—DEA Form 222
A DEA Form 222 is used to order Schedule II medications from a wholesaler or to transfer them to another pharmacy.

29. d—Perpetual inventory
A perpetual inventory shows the actual amount of a specific medication on hand in a pharmacy at any given moment.

30. a—Schedule II
A Schedule II medication may be partially filled for up to 60 days from the date of issuance for long-term care facility patients or individuals who are terminally ill. A long-term care facility may not have a DEA number assigned to it and therefore it cannot transfer a Schedule II medication back to the dispensing pharmacy.

31. d—Schedule V
A Schedule V medication is considered an exempt narcotic.

32. a—1
Only one 4-oz bottle of an exempt narcotic can be purchased in 48 hours.

33. b—18
An individual must be 18 years of age to purchase a bottle of an exempt narcotic.

34. b—DEA Form 41
A DEA Form 41 is used to request the destruction of controlled substances in a pharmacy. A retail pharmacy may have one destruction a year; however, a hospital may have "blanket destructions" for controlled substances.

35. e—5
The Controlled Substance Act consists of 5 schedules.

36. e—b and c only
There are two criteria to determine if a drug is placed in a particular drug schedule: (1) Does this medication have an approved medical use in the United States? (2) Does this medication cause either physical or psychological dependency?

37. c—10
The maximum number of different drugs that can be ordered on one DEA Form 222 are 10. There are no maximum quantities of a Schedule II medication that can be ordered at one time.

38. d—Place the form in the pharmacy safe and retain it. Use a new order form and write the order
If an error is made when completing a DEA Form 222 it must be retained in its entirety (all three copies) with the pharmacy records and a new DEA

Form 222 completed. Any alteration or erasure to a DEA Form 222 may result in the form being returned to the issuing pharmacy.

39. c—A medical doctor with a DEA number
A medical doctor with a DEA number may prescribe controlled substances.

40. c—1 week
A pharmacy that has accepted an emergency prescription for a Schedule II medication must receive a handwritten prescription from the prescriber within 1 week of the date it was called in to the pharmacy. Failure to do so may result in the prescriber being referred to the DEA.

41. a—I
Heroin is a Schedule I medication. It does not have an approved medical use in the United States. Heroin may cause both physical and psychological dependency.

42. a—0
A prescriber cannot write refills on a Schedule II medication.

43. f—5
A physician can authorize up to five refills for a Schedule III medication that must be used within 6 months from the date the prescription was written.

44. c—FDCA 1938
The enactment of the Food, Drug and Cosmetic Act of 1938 resulted in the formation of the Food and Drug Administration.

45. c—FDCA 1938
The failure to label a medication properly is an example of misbranding and was clearly defined under the Food, Drug and Cosmetic Act of 1938.

46. a—Ethics
The pharmacy technician's code of ethics states that a pharmacy technician is expected to remain competent.

47. c—FDCA 1938
Dispensing a medication in a dirty container is an example of adulteration. Adulteration was clearly defined in the Food, Drug and Cosmetic Act of 1938.

48. a—Ethics
A pharmacy technician is betraying a patient's trust by discussing his or her medical situation with an unauthorized person. This is a violation of the pharmacy technician's code of ethics, by which a technician is expected to keep all patient information confidential.

49. b—Pure Food and Drug Act of 1906
The Pure Food and Drug Act of 1906 was enacted as a result of the interstate transportation of adulterated and misbranded food and drug products.

50. c—FDCA 1938
The Food, Drug and Cosmetic Act of 1938 required that a New Drug Application be submitted before a drug entity could be approved by the FDA.

51. a—Ethics
    Ethics are being violated if an individual fails to ensure the health and safety of his or her patients.
52. f—5
    A physician can authorize up to five refills for a Schedule IV medication that must be used within 6 months from the date the prescription was written.
53. d—All of the above
    A prescription for a Schedule III medication may be handwritten by the physician and presented to the pharmacy by either the patient or the patient's representative, telephoned in to the pharmacy from the physician's office by a designated person, or faxed to the pharmacy from the physician's office.
54. c—6 months from the date the prescription was written
    A prescription for any controlled substance in Schedules III–V becomes void 6 months after the date it was written by the physician; it is not 6 months from the date it was originally filled.
55. d—All of the above
    A partial filling for a medication in Schedules III–V is permitted. However, the following conditions must be met: each filling is recorded in a similar manner as a refilling, the total quantity dispensed in partial fillings does not exceed the total quantity prescribed, no partial fillings occur after 6 months after the date the prescription was written, and a refill must be indicated on the prescription.

Acronyms

CMS—Centers for Medicare and Medicaid Services
DEA—Drug Enforcement Administration
DUE—Drug Utilization Evaluation
EPA—Environmental Protection Agency
FDA—Food and Drug Administration
HIPAA—Health Insurance Portability and Accountability Act
INDA—Investigational New Drug Application
NABP—National Association of Boards of Pharmacy
NDA—New Drug Application
NDC—National Drug Code
OSHA—Occupational Safety and Health Administration
TJC—The Joint Commission

Apply Your Knowledge Answers

1. The pharmacy may transfer this prescription and all remaining refills to another pharmacy. The transferring pharmacy must record the name, telephone number, address, and DEA number of the receiving pharmacy. The following other information must be included: the name of the receiving party, the date of the transfer, the number of units or refills remaining on the prescription, and the DEA number of the pharmacy. You must write "VOID" on your hard copy of the prescription. The prescription can be transferred only one time and it must be within 6 months of the date the prescription was written.
2. The patient may have the prescription filled for 15 tablets but he or she will not be able to receive the remaining quantity because the physician did not allow for a refill on the prescription.
3. Have the patient sign the back of the prescription to show he or she has requested ez open packaging.
4. Inform the patient of the situation. Your options are to order the medication or attempt to locate it at another pharmacy. If the medication is being ordered for the patient, you may dispense the 50 tablets in stock to the patient and provide the remaining tablets within 72 hours. If you are unable to have the remaining medication within 72 hours, the remaining quantity becomes void and at that time the physician should be notified of the situation.
5. Notify the pharmacist immediately. The pharmacist will make the decision on how to proceed.
6. Inform the patient that you must wait until the pharmacist returns to the pharmacy. An exempt narcotic can be dispensed only under the supervision of a pharmacist.
7. Inform the patient that you will ask the pharmacist for a recommendation when he or she is done talking on the phone. Inform the pharmacist of the situation and allow him or her to make the recommendation.
8. No, you should not inform the patient of the situation. It may appear that you are providing poor customer service; however, you are violating HIPAA by doing so. Only the owner of the prescription has the authority to authorize another individual to pick up the prescription.
9.
    a. Option 1 (three separate files)
       - A file for Schedule II drugs only
       - A file for Schedules III, IV, and V drugs only
       - A file for all non-controlled drugs
    b. Option 2 (two separate files)
       - A file for Schedule II drugs only
       - A file for all other prescriptions (Schedules III, IV, V, and non-controlled drugs); Schedules III, IV, and V must be stamped with a red "C"
    c. Option 3 (two separate files)
       - A file for all controlled prescriptions (Schedules III, IV, and V drugs must be stamped with a red "C")
       - A file for all non-controlled prescriptions
10. Heroin does not have an approved medical use in the United States.

Practice Your Knowledge Answers

Prescription #1. The physician has not included his or her DEA number on this prescription. Contact the physician's office to verify the prescription. Presently, federal law is being reviewed that will allow a pharmacy to add a missing DEA number to a prescription for a Schedule II medication. Until such time a decision is made, pharmacists must follow their state law.

Prescription #2. The prescription is a Schedule IV medication and must be filled within 6 months from the date it is written. Second, this medication can be refilled a maximum of five times. The pharmacy can contact the physician to seek permission for the prescription to be filled. If approved, the prescription must be rewritten as a new prescription and the old prescription disposed.

Prescription #3. The prescriber did not write the date on the prescription and wrote more than the approved number of refills (5). The pharmacy needs to contact the prescriber to obtain the date the prescription was written and verify the number of refills.

Prescription #4. Oxycontin is a Schedule II medication and cannot be refilled according to federal law. The pharmacist should be notified of the problem with the prescription. Often a pharmacist will contact the prescriber to verify the prescription has been written. If the prescription has been obtained fraudulently, the prescriber will instruct the pharmacist what to do. If the refill was written in error, the pharmacist should inform the patient of the situation.

Calculation Corner Answers

AS0123478: Add the first, third, and fifth numbers. Next add the second, fourth, and sixth numbers and multiply the sum by two. Then add the sum of the first set of numbers to the product of the second set of numbers. The number in the one's column should be the last number.

$$(0 + 2 + 4) = 6$$
$$(1 + 3 + 7)(2) = 22$$
$$6 + 22 = 28$$

The last number in the DEA number should be an 8.

BC2223333: Add the first, third, and fifth numbers. Next add the second, fourth, and sixth numbers and multiply the sum by two. Then add the sum of the first set of numbers to the product of the second set of numbers. The number in the one's column should be the last number.

$$(2 + 2 + 3) = 7$$
$$(2 + 3 + 3)(2) = 16$$
$$7 + 16 = 23$$

The last number in the DEA number should be a 3.

FD7654329: Add the first, third, and fifth numbers. Next add the second, fourth, and sixth numbers and multiply the sum by two. Then add the sum of the first set of numbers to the product of the second set of numbers. The number in the one's column should be the last number.

$$(7 + 5 + 3) = 15$$
$$(6 + 4 + 2)(2) = 24$$
$$15 + 24 = 39$$

The last number in the DEA number should be a 9.

MM1221593: Add the first, third, and fifth numbers. Next add the second, fourth, and sixth numbers and multiply the sum by two. Then add the sum of the first set of numbers to the product of the second set of numbers. The number in the one's column should be the last number.

$$(1 + 2 + 5) = 8$$
$$(2 + 1 + 9)(2) = 24$$
$$8 + 24 = 33$$

The last number in the DEA number should be a 3.

AZ3467025: Add the first, third, and fifth numbers. Next add the second, fourth, and sixth numbers and multiply the sum by two. Then add the sum of the first set of numbers to the product of the second set of numbers. The number in the one's column should be the last number.

$$(3 + 6 + 0) = 9$$
$$(4 + 7 + 2)(2) = 26$$
$$9 + 26 = 35$$

The last number in the DEA number should be a 5.

Pharmacy Facts—Research Answers

Table 4-1

Brand Name	Generic Name	Strengths	Schedule	List Two Indications of the Medication	List Three Adverse Effects of the Medication
Ativan	lorazepam	0.5, 1, & 2 mg	IV	Indications will vary	Adverse effects will vary
Dalmane	flurazepam	15 & 30 mg	IV	Indications will vary	Adverse effects will vary
Darvocet N 100	propoxyphene with acetaminophen	100/650 mg	IV	Indications will vary	Adverse effects will vary
Darvon 65	propoxyphene	65 mg	IV	Indications will vary	Adverse effects will vary

(Continued)

Table 4-1 (Continued)

Brand Name	Generic Name	Strengths	Schedule	List Two Indications of the Medication	List Three Adverse Effects of the Medication
Demerol	meperidine	10, 25, 50, 75, & 100 mg	II	Indications will vary	Adverse effects will vary
Dilaudid	hydromorphone	1, 2, 3, 4, 6, 8, 12, 18, 24, 30, & 32 mg	II	Indications will vary	Adverse effects will vary
Fiorcet	butalbital/ acetaminophen/ caffeine/codeine	50/325/40/ 30 mg	III	Indications will vary	Adverse effects will vary
Fiorinal	Butalbital/aspirin/ caffeine/codeine	50/325/40/ 30 mg	III	Indications will vary	Adverse effects will vary
Halcion	triazolam	0.125 & 0.25 mg	IV	Indications will vary	Adverse effects will vary
Librium	chlordiazepoxide	5, 10, & 25 mg	IV	Indications will vary	Adverse effects will vary
Lortab	hydrocodone/ acetaminophen	2.5/500 mg, 5/500 mg, 7.5/500 mg, & 10/500 mg	III	Indications will vary	Adverse effects will vary
Oxycontin	oxycodone	40 mg	II	Indications will vary	Adverse effects will vary
Percocet	oxycodone and acetaminophen	5 mg/325 mg	II	Indications will vary	Adverse effects will vary
Percodan	oxycodone and aspirin	5 mg/325 mg	II	Indications will vary	Adverse effects will vary
Restoril	temazepam	15 & 30 mg	IV	Indications will vary	Adverse effects will vary
Ritalin	methylphenidate	5, 10, 20, & 20 mg SR	II	Indications will vary	Adverse effects will vary
Robitussin AC	guaifenesin/codeine	100/10 mg per 5 mL	IV	Indications will vary	Adverse effects will vary
Stadol NS	butorphanol	2 & 10 mg	IV	Indications will vary	Adverse effects will vary
Tranxene	clorazepate	3.75, 7.5, 11.25, 15.0, & 22.5 mg	IV	Indications will vary	Adverse effects will vary
Tussionex	hydrocodone/ chlorpheniramine	10/8 mg per 5 mL	III	Indications will vary	Adverse effects will vary
Tylenol with Codeine	acetaminophen with codeine	325/15 mg, 325/30 mg, & 325/60 mg	III	Indications will vary	Adverse effects will vary
Tylox	oxycodone with acetaminophen	5/500 mg	II	Indications will vary	Adverse effects will vary
Valium	diazepam	2, 5, & 10 mg	IV	Indications will vary	Adverse effects will vary
Vicodin	hydrocodone with acetaminophen	5/500 mg, 7.5/750 mg, & 10/650 mg	III	Indications will vary	Adverse effects will vary
Vicoprofen	hydrocodone with acetaminophen	7.5 mg/200 mg	III	Indications will vary	Adverse effects will vary
Xanax	alprazolam	0.5, 1, 2, & 3 mg	IV	Indications will vary	Adverse effects will vary

Chapter 5 Lab

Multiple Choice Answers

1. c—12/20

   12/20 can be reduced to 3/5 by dividing both the numerator and the denominator by 4 which makes these two fractions equivalent.

   Numerator $\quad 12 \div 4 = 3$
   Denominator $\quad 20 \div 4 = 5$

2. b—14/16

   14/16 can be reduced to 7/8 by dividing both the numerator and the denominator by 2 which makes these two fractions equivalent.

   Numerator $\quad 14 \div 2 = 7$
   Denominator $\quad 16 \div 2 = 8$

3. a—0.375
   A fraction can be converted to a decimal by dividing the numerator by the denominator.
   $3 \div 8 = 0.375$

4. d—0.133.
   A fraction can be converted to a decimal by dividing the numerator by the denominator.
   $2 \div 15 = 0.133$

5. a—40%
   A fraction can be converted to a percent by dividing the numerator by the denominator and multiplying by 100 and adding the percent sign.
   $2 \div 5 = 0.4$
   $0.4 \times 100 = 40\%$

6. b—41.67%
   A fraction can be converted to a percent by dividing the numerator by the denominator and multiplying by 100 and adding the percent sign.
   $5 \div 12 = 0.4167$
   $0.4167 \times 100 = 41.67\%$

7. a—2/15
   Multiplication of fractions is accomplished by multiplying numerator-by-numerator and denominator-by-denominator; then reduce the problem to lowest terms.
   $\frac{1}{3} \times \frac{2}{5} = \frac{2}{15}$

8. c—3/8
   Multiplication of fractions is accomplished by multiplying numerator-by-numerator and denominator-by-denominator; then reduce the problem to lowest terms.
   $\frac{3}{4} \times \frac{1}{2} = \frac{3}{8}$

9. b—5/6
   Division of two fractions is accomplished by inverting the second fraction, change the division sign to a multiplication sign, and multiply the two fractions.
   $\frac{2}{3} \times \frac{5}{4} = \frac{10}{12}$
   This can be reduced to 5/6 by dividing both by 2.

10. c—7.5 mL
    You must know conversions between the household system and the metric system.
    1 tsp = 5 mL
    1.5×5 mL = 7.5 mL

11. b—4 tbsp
    You must know conversions between the household system and the metric system.
    1 tbsp = 15 mL
    (60 mL $\div$ 15 mL) $\times$ 1 tbsp = 4 tbsp

12. d—2.5 fl oz
    You must know conversions between the household system and the metric system.

1 fl oz = 30 mL
(75 mL $\div$ 30 mL) $\times$ 1 fl oz = 2.5 fl oz

13. c—2500 mL
    You must know the metric system to convert liters to milliliters. Multiply the number of liters by 1000.
    $2.5 \times 1000 = 2500$ mL

14. a—0.23 kg
    You must know the metric system to convert grams to kilograms. Divide the number of grams by 1000.
    230 g $\div$ 1000 = 0.23 kg

15. c—82.4°F
    Problem can be solved using the following formula:
    $9°C = 5°F - 160$

16. a—12.7°C
    Problem can be solved using the following formula:
    $9°C = 5°F - 160$

17. a—0.5 tablet
    (25 mg $\div$ 50 mg) $\times$ 1 tablet = 0.5 tablet

18. d—2 tablets
    Convert grams to milligrams:
    0.5 g $\times$ 1000 = 500 mg
    (500 mg $\div$ 250 mg) $\times$ 1 tablet = 2 tablets

19. a—0.5 mL
    Convert grams to milligrams:
    1 g = 60 mg
    60 mg $\times$ 0.25 = 15 mg
    (15 mg $\div$ 30 mg) $\times$ 1 mL = 0.5 mL

20. c—9 mL
    (225 mg $\div$ 125 mg) $\times$ 5 mL = 9 mL

21. d—3 tsp
    1 tsp = 5 mL
    (75 mg $\div$ 25 mg) $\times$ 1 tsp = 3 tsp

22. b—0.4 mL
    (0.8 mg $\div$ 2 mg) $\times$ 1 mL = 0.4 mL

23. d—1.6 mL
    (40 mg $\div$ 25 mg) $\times$ 1 mL = 1.6 mL

24. b—75 mg
    Clark's Rule = [(Weight of individual in pounds)/150 pounds] $\times$ Adult dose
    $\frac{45}{150} \times 250$ mg = 75 mg

25. a—30 mg
    Clark's Rule = [(Weight of individual in pounds)/150 pounds] $\times$ Adult dose
    $\frac{60}{150} \times 75$ mg = 30 mg

26. d—100 mg

    Clark's Rule = [(Weight of individual in pounds)/150 pounds] × Adult dose

    $$\frac{75}{150} \times 200 \text{ mg} = 100 \text{ mg}$$

27. c—60 mg

    Young's Rule = [(Age in years)/(Age in years + 12)] × Adult dose

    $$\frac{8}{8 + 12 = 20} \times 150 \text{ mg} = 60 \text{ mg}$$

28. a—15 mg

    Young's Rule = [(Age in years)/(Age in years + 12)] × Adult dose

    $$\frac{5}{5 + 12 = 17} \times 50 \text{ mg} = 15 \text{ mg}$$

29. b—25 mL of the 10% solution

    This is a dilution problem and can be solved using the following formula:

    (Initial strength × Initial volume) = (Final strength × Final volume)
    (10% × IV) = (2.5% × 100 mL)

    $$\frac{2.5\% \times 100 \text{ mL}}{10\%} = 25 \text{ mL}$$

30. a—20 mL of the 30% solution

    This is a dilution problem and can be solved using the following formula:

    (Initial strength × Initial volume) = (Final strength × Final volume)
    (30% × IV) = (1.2% × 500 mL)

    $$\frac{1.2\% \times 500 \text{ mL}}{30\%} = 20 \text{ mL}$$

31. c—200 mL of 1% + 250 mL of 10%

    Alligation problem:

    ```
    10          5     (5 ÷ 9) = (0.556 × 450 mL)
          6                   = 250 mL of 10%
     1          4     (4 ÷ 9) = (0.444 × 450 mL)
    _____                  = 200 mL of 1%
          9
    ```

32. d—75 mL of 1% + 25 mL of 3%

    Alligation problem:

    ```
     3          0.5   (0.5 ÷ 2) = (0.25 × 100 mL)
          1.5                   = 25 mL of 3%
     1          1.5   (1.5 ÷ 2) = (0.75 × 100 mL)
    _____                    = 75 mL of 1%
          2.0
    ```

33. b—125 mL/h

    This is a flow rate problem and can be solved by dividing the volume (V) by the time (T):

    1000 mL (V) ÷ 8 h (T) = 125 mL/h

34. c—83 mL/h

    This is a flow rate problem and can be solved by dividing the volume (V) by the time (T):

    500 mL (V) ÷ 6 h (T) = 83 mL/h

35. c—150 mL/h

    This is a flow rate problem and can be solved by dividing the volume (V) by the time (T):

    1800 mL (V) ÷ 12 h (T) = 150 mL/h

36. b—125 gtts/min

    This is a flow rate problem and can be solved by using the following formula:

    (Rate × Drop factor) ÷ (Time conversion) = Drops per minute
    (250 mL × 15 gtts/mL) ÷ 30 min = 125 gtts/min

37. a—21 gtts/min

    This is a flow rate problem and can be solved by using the following formula:

    (Rate × Drop factor) ÷ (Time conversion) = Drops per minute

    Convert liters to milliliters:

    0.5 L × 1000 = 500 mL

    Convert hours to minutes:

    1 h = 60 min
    60 min × 6 = 360 min
    (500 mL × 15 gtts/mL) ÷ 360 min = 20.83 gtts/min; round up to 21 gtts/min

38. d—100 gtts/min

    This is a flow rate problem and can be solved by using the following formula:

    (Rate × Drop factor) ÷ (Time conversion) = Drops per minute
    Microdrip tubing = 60 gtts/mL

    Convert hours to minutes:

    1 h = 60 min
    60 min × 10 = 600 min
    (1000 mL × 60 gtts/mL) ÷ 600 min = 100 gtts/min

39. b—0.72 g

    30 mg × 24 h = 720 mg

    Convert milligrams to grams:

    720 mg ÷ 1000 = 0.72 g

40. c—25 gtts/min

    This is a flow rate problem and can be solved by using the following formula:

    (Rate × Drop factor) ÷ (Time conversion) = Drops per minute

    Convert hours to minutes:

1 h = 60 min
60 min × 12 = 720 min
(1800 mL × 10 gtts/mL) ÷ 720 min = 25 gtts/min

41.

mL	tsp	tbsp	fl oz	cup	pt	qt	gal
3840	768	256	128	16	8	4	1
960	192	64	32	4	2	1	0.25
480	96	32	16	2	1	0.5	0.125
240	48	16	8	1	0.5	0.25	0.0625
960							
	96						
720	144	48	24	3	1.5	0.75	0.1875
			16				
1440	288	96	48	8	4	2	0.5
4800	960	320	160	20	10	5	1.25
7680	1536	512	256	32	16	8	2
							2

Apply Your Knowledge Answers

1. 6.5 tablets

   1 g = 65 mg
   65 mg × 30 = 1950 mg

   Convert milligrams to grams:

   1000 mg = 1 g
   1950 mg ÷ 1000 = 1.95 g
   (1.95 g ÷ 0.3 g) × 1 tablet = 6.5 tablets

2. 200 g

   If each bottle contains 50 mL and you need 100 bottles:

   50 mL × 100 = 5000 mL

   Divide by 2.5 mL:

   5000 mL ÷ 2.5 mL = 2000

   Multiple by strength per 2.5 mL:

   2000 × 100 mg = 200,000 mg

   Convert milligrams to grams:

   200,000 mg ÷ 1000 = 200 g

3. Salicylic acid, 4.54 g
   Menthol, 1.135 g
   There are 453.5924 g in a pound.

   1 g/100 g = 1%
   453.5924 ÷ 100 = 4.54
   Salicylic acid, 4.54 g
   1% = 4.539
   ¼% = 1 ÷ 4 = 0.25
   4.539 × 0.25 = 1.135
   Menthol, 1.135 g

4. 300 mg
   Convert pounds to kilograms:

   1 lb = 2.2 kg
   132 ÷ 2.2 = 60 kg
   5 mg × 60 = 300 mg

5. 4.5 gal

   1 gal = 128 oz
   144 × 4 oz = 576 oz
   (576 oz ÷ 128 oz) × 1 gal = 4.5 gal

6. 3.75 mL
   Convert pounds to kilograms:

   1 lb = 2.2 kg
   165 lb ÷ 2.2 = 75 kg
   25 mcg × 75 = 1875 mcg
   (1875 mcg ÷ 500 mcg) × 1 mL = 3.75 mL

7. 18.91 mL
   Convert pounds to kilograms:

   52 lb ÷ 2.2 = 23.64 kg
   23.64 × 400,000 units = 9,456,000 units
   (9,456,000 units ÷ 500,000 units) × 1 mL
   = 18.91 mL

8. 100 mL

   (Initial strength × Initial volume) = (Final strength × Final volume)
   (20% × IV) = (5% × 400 mL)

   $$\frac{5\% \times 400\ mL}{20\%} = 100\ mL$$

9. 523 g
   Convert 1 cup to milliliters:

   8 oz = 1 cup
   1 oz = 30 mL
   30 mL × 8 = 240 mL
   1.25 g × 240 = 300 g
   0.93 g × 240 = 223 g
   300 g + 223 g = 523 g

10. 1.5 mg

    0.025 × 60 = 1.5

11. 400 mL

12. 93.5 mL

    (Initial strength × Initial volume) = (Final strength × Final volume)
    1:8 = 1 ÷ 8 = 0.125
    1:6 = 1 ÷ 6 = 0.167

    $$\frac{125\ mL \times 0.125}{0.167} = 93.5\ mL$$

13. 18.75 mL

    (Initial strength × Initial volume) = (Final strength × Final volume)
    1:4 = 1 ÷ 4 = 0.25

$2:5 = 2 \div 5 = 0.40$

$$\frac{30 \text{ mL} \times 0.25}{0.40} = 18.75 \text{ mL}$$

14. 1.78 mL

   (Initial strength $\times$ Initial volume) = (Final strength $\times$ Final volume)

   Convert 14% to a decimal:

   $14\% \div 100 = 0.14$

   Convert 1:4 to a decimal:

   $1:4 = 1 \div 4 = 0.25$

   Convert liters to milliliters:

   1 L = 1000 mL

   $$\frac{1000 \text{ mL} \times 0.25}{0.14} = 1.78 \text{ mL}$$

15. 186.67 mL

   (Initial strength $\times$ Initial volume) = (Final strength $\times$ Final volume)

   Convert 1:5 to a decimal:

   $1:5 = 1 \div 5 = 0.20$

   Convert 30% to a decimal:

   $30\% \div 100 = 0.30$

   $$\frac{280 \text{ mL} \times 0.20}{0.30} = 186.66 \text{ mL; round up to } 186.67 \text{ mL}$$

16. 14.28%

   (Initial strength $\times$ Initial volume) = (Final strength $\times$ Final volume)

   120 mL + 300 mL = 420 mL

   $$\frac{120 \text{ mL} \times 50\%}{420 \text{ mL}} = 14.28 \%$$

17. 1000 g

   1 g/100 g = 1%
   10 g/X = 1%
   1 g $\times$ 10 g = 10 g
   100 g $\times$ 10 g = 1000 g

18. 0.1%

   1 g/100 mL = 1.0%
   $1 \div 100 = 0.01 \times 100\% = 1\%$
   0.5 g $\div$ 500 mL = 0.1%
   0.5 g $\div$ 500 mL = 0.001 $\times$ 100% = 0.1%

19. 400 g

25		5	$(5 \div 25) = (0.20 \times 500 \text{ g})$
	5		= 100 g of 25%
0		20	$(20 \div 25) = (0.80 \times 500 \text{ g})$
	25		= 400 g of generic ointment

20. You would use 72 mL of the 5% solution and 48 mL of distilled water.

5		3	$(3 \div 5) = (0.60 \times 120 \text{ mL})$
	3		= 72 mL of 5% solution
0		2	$(2 \div 5) = (0.40 \times 120 \text{ mL})$
	5		= 48 mL of distilled water

21. You would use 62.5 mL of the 25% solution and 37.5 mL of the 65% solution.

65		15	$(15 \div 40) = (0.375 \times 100 \text{ mL})$
	40		= 37.5 mL of 65% solution
25		25	$(25 \div 40) = (0.635 \times 100 \text{ mL})$
	40		= 62.5 mL of 25% solution

22. You would use 50 g of the 10% and 40 g of the 1% ointment.

10		1	$(1 \div 9) = (0.111 \times 45 \text{ g})$
	2		= 50 g of 10% ointment
1		8	$(8 \div 9) = (0.888 \times 45 \text{ g})$
	9		= 40 g of 1% ointment

23. You would use 42.9 mL of the 7.5% solution and 57.1 mL of the 1:200 solution.
   Convert 1:200 to a percent:

   $1:200 = (1 \div 200) = (0.005 \times 100\%) = 0.50$

7.5		3	$(3 \div 7) = (0.429 \times 100 \text{ mL})$
	3.5		= 42.9 g of 7.5% solution
0.5		4	$(4 \div 7) = (0.571 \times 100 \text{ mL})$
	7		= 57.1 g of 1:200 solution

24. 3 tablets

   (Initial strength $\times$ Initial volume) = (Final strength $\times$ Final volume)

   (100 mg $\times$ IV) = (20 mg/mL $\times$ 150 mL) = 300 mg

   $$\frac{20 \text{ mg/mL} \times 150 \text{ mL}}{100 \text{ mg}}$$

   (300 mg $\div$ 100 mg) $\times$ 1 tablet = 3 tablets

25. 1%

   1 g/100 mL = 1.0%
   $1 \div 100 = 0.01 \times 100\% = 1\%$
   2.4/240 mL = 1%
   2.4 g $\div$ 240 mL = 0.01 $\times$ 100% = 1%

26. It would take 5 hours to infuse. The flow rate is 4 gtts/min.

   75 mL $\div$ 15 mL = 5
   5 $\times$ 60 min = 300 min
   (75 mL $\times$ 15 gtts/min) $\div$ 300 min = 3.75 gtts/min; round to 4 gtts/min

27. 60 gtts/min

    10,000 units ÷ 80 units/min = 125 min
    500 mL × 15 gtts/mL = 7500 gtts
    7500 gtts ÷ 125 min = 60 gtts/min

28. The pharmacy would need to send three 1-L bags to the nursing unit.

    1 L = 1000 mL
    100 mL × 24 = 2400 mL
    Three 1-L bags are needed.

29. The next bag should be started at 0100 hours on Thursday.

    1000 mL ÷ 100 mL/h = 10 h
    1500 hours = 3:00 pm
    3:00 pm + 10 hours = 1:00 am or 0100 hours

30. The IV should be infused at a rate of 41.67 mL/h and it will take 12 h to infuse the entire 500-mL bag.

    12% = 12 g/100 mL
    500 mL ÷ 100 mL = 5
    12 g × 5 = 60 g/500 mL
    60 g ÷ 5 g = 12

    It will take 12 hours to infuse.

    500 mL ÷ 12 h = 41.667 mL/h; round to 41.7

    The rate will be 41.67 mL/h.

31. 500 mL

    1100 hours = 11:00 am
    2100 hours = 9:00 pm
    Total infusion time = 10 h
    50 mL × 10 h = 500 mL

32. 5.76 L

    1 L = 1000 mL
    60 mL × 96 h = 5760 mL
    5760 mL ÷ 1000 = 5.76 L

33. 78 mL/h

    (20 gtts/min ÷ 15 gtts/mL) = 1.3 mL/min
    1.3 mL/min × 60 min = 78 mL/h

34. 20 gtts/mL

    66 gtts/min × 60 min = 3960 gtts/h
    1000 mL ÷ 5 h = 200 mL/h
    3960 gtts/h ÷ 200 mL/h = 19.80 gtts/mL; round to 20 gtts/mL

35. 11.25 mEq/h

    500 mL ÷ 125 mL/h = 4 h
    45 mEq ÷ 4 h = 11.25 mEq/h

Practice Your Knowledge Answers

Which method of calculation is best for this child and why? Young's Rule is used to calculate a dose based on a child's age in years:

Young's Rule = [(Age in years)/(Age in years +12] × Adult dose
11/(11 +12) × 500 mg = 239 mg

Clark's Rule is used to calculate a dose based on weight:

Clark's Rule = [(Weight in pounds)/150 pounds] × Adult dose
95/150 × 500 mg = 316 mg

Body surface area (BSA) is calculated using a nomogram. Draw a straight line from 95 lb to 62 in. The line intersects the body surface at 1.36:

(BSA/1.7 × Adult dose) = Dose given
(1.36/1.7) × 500 mg = 400 mg

Using body surface area is the most accurate method of calculation because it takes into consideration both the weight and height of the child.

Calculation Corner Answers

Solution

How much of each ingredient will you need to prepare this compound? You are making less than the original formula calls for and therefore you will need to reduce the formula.

Quantity to make/Original formula = Reducing factor
240 mL/1000 mL = 0.24

Multiply the quantity in the original formula by 0.24:

Calamine	80 g × 0.24 = 19.2 g
Zinc oxide	80 g × 0.24 = 19.2 g
Glycerin	20 g × 0.24 = 4.8 g
Bentonite magma	250 mL × 0.24 = 60 mL
Calcium hydroxide sol qs	1000 mL × 0.24 = 240 mL

Chapter 6 Lab
Multiple Choice Answers

1. d—All of the above
   Some of the factors that can affect the absorption of a medication include the patient's age, health condition, and the presence of food in the digestive system.
2. d—All of the above
   The kidneys are the primary organ involved with the elimination of a drug from the body; however, the lungs and skin can also eliminate the drug from the body.
3. b—Bioavailability is defined by federal regulations as the rate and extent to which the active ingredient or active moiety is absorbed from a drug product and becomes available at the site of action

Bioavailability is the rate and the extent by which an active ingredient is absorbed from a drug product and becomes available at the site of action to produce a therapeutic effect.

4. c—FDA

   The FDA assigns a nonproprietary name to a medication; the drug manufacturer assigns a proprietary name.

5. d—All of the above

   The following factors can affect the absorption of a medication: drug solubility, drug disintegration rate, drug concentration, blood flow to the absorption site, and the size of the absorbing surface area.

6. d—All of the above

   A drug may accumulate in plasma proteins, fat, extracellular areas, cellular areas, and in some cases in muscle tissue. A medication may also build up in intracellular areas and the liver.

7. d—All of the above

   The metabolic processes of oxidation, reduction, and hydrolysis use nonmicrosomal enzymes.

8. c—Passive glomerular filtration

   The kidney eliminates a drug and its metabolites through glomerular filtration, active tubular secretions, and passive tubular reabsorption. A drug does not undergo passive glomerular filtration during its elimination from the body.

9. d—All of the above

   The cell membrane and its components on either side of the membrane may or may not allow a drug to cross it. Depending on whether a drug is a weak acid or base will have an effect on the ionized and unionized forms of a drug will cross the cell membrane. Unionized drugs are lipid soluble and are able to easily cross the cell membrane. Ionized forms of a drug have difficulty crossing the lipid membrane because of its low lipid solubility or size. Most medications cross the cell membrane through passive transport, which requires no energy to be used by the substance. On the other hand, active transport is extremely selective in nature and requires energy.

10. d—Homeostasis

    Homeostasis is not a factor that affects a drug's absorption. The following factors do affect a drug's absorption: solubility, disintegration, concentration, blood flow, and surface area.

11. c—Chemically equivalent

    Chemically equivalent agents must meet both chemical and physical standards established by governmental and regulatory agencies. Bioavailability refers to the rate and extent to which an active drug is absorbed into the body. The FDA oversees bioavailability testing on all medications. Biologically equivalent medications have similar concentrations in the blood and tissue. Therapeutically equivalent medications provide the same therapeutic effect. The USP establishes therapeutic equivalent codes for medications.

12. b—AB

    Medications assigned a bioequivalence code of AB have met the necessary bioequivalence requirements. AA rated drugs are products that have been deemed therapeutically equivalent to other pharmaceutically equivalent products and have not demonstrated any bioequivalence problems. Medications designated AN are solutions and aerosols, while AO signifies injectable oil solutions; neither code demonstrates bioequivalence issues due to the dosage form.

13. a—B*

    Medications with a B*code need further FDA investigation and review.

14. c—Passive transport (diffusion)

    Passive transport (diffusion) is the process by which a substance goes from higher to lower concentration. Active transport is the process that requires energy and the drug goes from lower to higher concentration. Filtration is the process by which a drug is eliminated through the kidneys. This process is dependent on a substance's protein binding and glomerular filtration rate. Redistribution is the process by which a drug is reallocated from one site to another site. Redistribution is observed with many cardiovascular medications that are either injected intravenously or inhaled.

15. a—Pharmacognosy

    Pharmacognosy is the study and identification of natural products used as drugs. Pharmacology is the science that deals with the knowledge of the history of a drug; the source of a drug; the physical and chemical properties of a drug; the compounding of a drug; the biochemical and physiological effects of a drug; the mechanism of action of a drug; the absorption, distribution, biotransformation, and excretion of a drug; and the drug's therapeutic use. Pharmacodynamics is the response following administration of a drug that is directly related to its concentration of the drug at the site of its action. Pharmacokinetics is the study of the absorption, distribution, metabolism, and elimination of a drug.

16. d—Pharmacology is a science that deals with the dosage form of a drug

    Pharmacology does *not* deal with the dosage form of the drug. It is described fully in the answer to question 15 above.

17. b—Antagonism

    An antagonist is a drug that does not bind to a specific site and which prevents a drug from producing its effect. Addition is the combined effect of two drugs, where the sum of their effects is equal to each of them being taken alone. Potentiation is the process where one drug increases the potency or strength of another drug and the effect is greater than the effect of each drug prescribed alone. Synergism is a drug interaction where the combined effect of two drugs if taken together is greater than the sum of its parts.

18. b—Pregnancy Category B

Pregnancy Category B is assigned to drugs for which drug studies have not been performed in pregnant women and in which animal studies have not demonstrated fetal risk. Pregnancy Category A is awarded to medications for which drug studies in pregnant women have not demonstrated risk to the fetus. Pregnancy Category C means that drug studies have been performed in pregnant women or animals and have revealed some teratogenic potential but the risk to the fetus is unknown. Pregnancy Category NR indicates the drug has not been rated by the FDA.

19. c—Enzyme concentrations within the liver will increase resulting in an increase in drug metabolism

Liver enzyme concentrations decrease (not increase) within the liver as we age.

20. b—An individual will experience improved memory and learning functions

Behavioral toxicity results in decreased memory and learning functions, not improved memory and learning functions.

21. b—Antibiotics

Any medication that alters an individual's mood or perception demonstrates the potential to be abused and result in drug dependence. Antibiotics have not demonstrated a potential to be abused. Medications that have shown this potential include opioids, sedatives, alcohol, amphetamines, and CNS stimulants and depressants.

22. b—Physical dependence

Physical dependence is demonstrated when a medication is suddenly stopped or withdrawn from the patient resulting in physical symptoms appearing.

23. a—Buccal

A parenteral drug is one that bypasses the digestive system. A buccal tablet is placed between the gum and cheek; it does not avoid the digestive system.

24. a—Biologically equivalent

Biologically equivalent medications have similar concentrations in the blood and tissue. Chemically equivalent agents must meet both chemical and physical standards established by governmental and regulatory agencies. Therapeutically equivalent medications provide the same therapeutic effect. The USP establishes therapeutic equivalent codes for medications.

25. c—Potentiation

Potentiation is the process where one drug increases the potency or strength of another drug and the effect is greater than the effect of each drug prescribed alone. An antagonist is a drug that does not bind to a specific site and prevents a drug from producing its effect. Addition is the combined effect of two drugs, where the sum of their effects is equal to each of them being taken alone. Synergism is a drug interaction where the combined effect of two drugs if taken together is greater than the sum of its parts.

26. c—Metabolism

Metabolism is the process of converting a drug to a condition where it may be eliminated by the body. Absorption is the process by which the drug enters the bloodstream. Distribution is the process by which a medication reaches its site of action. Elimination is the process by which the drug is removed from the body.

27. a—Cardiac defects

Lithium is capable of crossing the placental barrier and may cause cardiac defects in the fetus.

28. a—Conjugation

Conjugation is a synthetic chemical reaction that occurs during a drug's metabolism. Hydrolysis, oxidation, and reduction are nonsynthetic reactions.

29. d—Pregnancy Category X

Pregnancy Category X designates that drug studies have revealed teratogenic effects in women and/or animals. The fetal risk outweighs the benefit of the drug and is contraindicated in pregnancy. Pregnancy Category A is awarded to those medications where drug studies in pregnant women have not been demonstrated a risk to the fetus. Pregnancy Category B is given to those drugs where drug studies have not been performed in pregnant women and animal studies have not demonstrated fetal risk. Pregnancy Category C means that drug studies have been performed in pregnant women or animals have revealed some teratogenic potential but the risk to the fetus is unknown.

30. c—Enzyme inhibition

Enzyme inhibition causes a decrease in the number of enzymes present in the body during metabolism.

True/False Answers

1. True.
2. False. It takes four to five half-lives for a drug to be eliminated from the body.
3. True.
4. True.
5. True.
6. True.
7. True.
8. True.
9. True.
10. True.
11. False. An idiosyncrasy is an unusual effect of a drug regardless of the intensity or dosage.
12. True.
13. False. Synergism is a drug interaction where the combined effect of the two drugs is greater than the sum of its parts.

14. True.
15. False. In most situations, medication should be taken on an empty stomach unless otherwise noted.

Acronyms

ADME—absorption, distribution, metabolism, elimination
CDC—Centers for Disease Control and Prevention
FDA—Food and Drug Administration
MTC—minimum toxic concentration
OTC—over-the-counter
USAN—United States Adopted Names
USP—United States Pharmacopeia

Apply Your Knowledge Answers

1. Nitroglycerin is available as a 0.3 mg, 0.4 mg and 0.6 mg sublingual tablet, a 20 mg, 40 mg, 60 mg, 80 mg, 120 mg and 160 transdermal system and 400 mcg lingual spray.
2. Answers will vary depending on the selection of the antibiotic.
3. Loading dose; The physician would use a loading dose to obtain a therapeutic level quicker in the body.
4. Maintenance dose.
5. Foods that are high in Vitamin K, such as romaine lettuce, spinach, kale and cabbage may interact with Coumadin.
6. A generic drug contains the same active ingredient in the same strength in the same dosage form taken in the same administration route as the brand name drug. A generic drug is available after the patent has expired.
7. The unborn child may develop birth defects as a result of a pregnant woman taking Accutane. Accutane crosses the placental barrier and therefore birth defects may occur.
8. The patient is probably undergoing caffeine withdrawal.
9.

Drug	Effect If Drug Concentration Is Below the Recommended Therapeutic Level	Effect If Drug Concentration Is Above the Recommended Therapeutic Level
Coumadin	Blood begins to clot and could result in possible embolism	Possible hemorrhage
Dilantin	Seizures may develop	Respiratory and circulatory depression
Lithium Carbonate	Dehydration	Lithium toxicity
Synthroid	Hypothyroidism	Hyperthyroidism

Practice Your Knowledge Answers

1.

Medication	Drug Interactions	Warnings
Advil	NSAIDs, warfarin	stomach bleeding, asthma, heart, drowsiness
Afrin Nasal Spray	none	heart problems, high blood pressure, thyroid disease, diabetes
Alka-Seltzer	aspirin, warfarin	asthma, ulcers, bleeding disorders
Bayer Aspirin	warfarin	Reyes Syndrome, pregnancy, ulcer
Benadryl	none	Glaucoma, breathing problems, emphysema, bronchitis, pregnancy
Chlor-Trimeton	none	Emphysema, bronchitis, glaucoma
Claritin	none	Liver or kidney disease, drowsiness, pregnancy
Cortaid	none	External use only,
Imodium AD	none	Pregnancy, bloody stools
Lotrimin	none	External use only
Melatonin	Alcohol	Do not drive or use machinery, pregnancy
Metamucil	none	None
Milk of Magnesia	none	Kidney disease, magnesium replacement therapy, nausea and vomiting
Mylanta	none	Kidney disease, magnesium replacement therapy
Neosporin	none	External use only
Pepcid AC	none	Pregnant, breast feeding, kidney disease, allergic to famotidine
Robitussin	MAOI	Drowsiness
St. John's Wort	none	Pregnancy, not to be taken by anyone under 18yrs of age
Sudafed	none	Heart disease, high blood pressure, thyroid disease, prostate
Tavist-D	none	Heart disease, high blood pressure, thyroid disease
Vicks Cough Syrup	MAOI	Asthma, emphysema, bronchitis
Vitron C	none	Only under supervision by physician, constipation, keep out of reach of children under the age of 6
Zostrix	none	External use, not to be used by anyone under the age of 18

Practice Your Knowledge Answers

2.

Medication	Active Ingredient	Available Dosage Forms	Routes of Administration
Advil	ibuprofen	Tablet, caplet and liquid-gels	Oral
Anusol	hydrocortisone	Cream, ointment and suppository	Topical
Bayer Aspirin	acetylsalicylic acid	Tablet	Oral
Benadryl	diphenhydramine	Capsule, gel tab, tablet, elixir and syrup	Oral and topical
Claritin	loratidine	Tablet, syrup	Oral
Comtrex	Acetaminophen/ dextromethorphan/ phenylephrine	Caplet	Oral
Cortaid	hydrocortisone	Cream and ointment	Topical
Dimetapp	brompheniramine	Tablet and syrup	Oral
Lotrimin	clotrimazole	Cream	Topical
Maalox	aluminum hydroxide/ magnesium hydroxide	Suspension and tablet	Oral
Mylanta	aluminum hydroxide/ magnesium hydroxide	Suspension and tablet	Oral
Neosporin	bacitracin/neomycin/ polymixin	Cream and ointment	Topical
Pepto Bismol	Bismuth subsalicylate	Suspension and tablet	Oral
Robitussin	guaifenesin	Syrup	Oral
Tylenol	acetaminophen	Tablet, caplet, gel tab, syrup, elixir, suspension, drops and suppository	Oral and rectal
Zyrtec	cetirizine	Tablet and syrup	Oral

Calculation Corner Answers

Solution

1. How much medication remains after four half-lives? A half-life is defined as the amount of time needed for 50% of the drug to be eliminated:

After the first half-life, 250 mg of drug is remaining
After the second half-life, 125 mg of drug is remaining
After the third half-life, 62.5 mg of drug is remaining
After the fourth half-life, 31.25 mg of drug is remaining

Pharmacy Facts—Research Answers

Table 6-1

Brand Name	Generic Name	List Five Adverse Effects	Nephrotoxicity (yes or no)	Hepatotoxicity (yes or no)	List Any Teratogenic Effects
Accutane	isotretinoin	Answers will vary	No	Yes	Fetal injury and birth defects
Achromycin	tetracycline	Answers will vary	No	No	Discoloration of teeth
Bactrim	Trimethoprim/ sulfamethoxazole	Answers will vary	Yes	No	Cleft palates
Cipro	ciprofloxacin	Answers will vary	No	No	Not established

(Continued)

Table 6-1 *(Continued)*

Brand Name	Generic Name	List Five Adverse Effects	Nephrotoxicity (yes or no)	Hepatotoxicity (yes or no)	List Any Teratogenic Effects
Coumadin	warfarin	Answers will vary	Yes	Yes	No
Diflucan	fluconazole	Answers will vary	No	Yes	No
Dilantin	phenytoin	Answers will vary	No	No	Congenital malformations
Epivir	lamivudine	Answers will vary	Yes	No	Not established
Eskalith	lithium carbonate	Answers will vary	Yes	No	Cardiac anomalies
Estrace	estradiol	Answers will vary	No	No	No
Garamycin	gentamycin	Answers will vary	Yes	Yes	No
Lamisil	terbinafine	Answers will vary	No	Yes	No
Minocin	minocycline	Answers will vary	No	No	Discoloration of teeth
Oxycontin	oxycodone	Answers will vary	Yes	Yes	No
Paxil	paroxetine	Answers will vary	No	No	Cardiovascular malformations
Ritalin	methylphenidate	Answers will vary	No	No	Not determined
Sporanox	itraconazole	Answers will vary	Possible	Yes	Not determined
Synthroid	levothyroxine	Answers will vary	No	No	No
Vancocin	vancomycin	Answers will vary	Yes	No	No
Vasotec	enalapril	Answers will vary	Yes	Yes	Fetal and neonatal morbidity
Vibramycin	doxycycline	Answers will vary	No	No	Tooth discoloration
Wellbutrin	bupropion	Answers will vary	Limited information	Yes	No
Yaz	Drospirenone/ ethinyl estradiol	Answers will vary	No	Yes	Medications containing estrogens should not be taken during pregnancy
Zestril	lisinopril	Answers will vary	Yes	Yes	Fetal and neonatal morbidity
Zithromax	azithromycin	Answers will vary	No	No	No testing has been done

Chapter 7 Lab
Multiple Choice Answers

1. c—Cimetidine
   Cimetidine is a histamine-2 receptor blocker. Minocycline and penicillin are categorized by antibacterial drug families (tetracycline and penicillin, respectively). Ibuprofen is also classified by the family to which it belongs, nonsteroidal anti-inflammatory drugs (NSAIDs).

2. d—Zolpidem
   Zolpidem is a sedative-hypnotic employed in the management of insomnia.

3. b—Contraindication
   A contraindication means that the medication should not be administered under specified circumstances. An indication is the approved use for the medication, while a drug interaction indicates the pharmacodynamics of administering more than one drug at a time.

4. c—Alprazolam
    Alprazolam is a benzodiazepine, sedative-hypnotic agent that is used in the management of anxiety and insomnia.

5. c—Methamphetamine
    Penicillin is a antibiotic, Codeine is a scheduled drug but not illicit, and Ambien is a sleeping medication.

6. b—Prempro
    Prempro is not an oral contraceptive, but constitutes hormonal replacement therapy (HRT) and is usually give to postmenopausal women.

7. b—Omeprazole
    Heparin is an anticoagulant agent, albuterol is a bronchodilator, and adderal is used to treat ADHD.

8. a—Timolol
    Timolol is a beta adrenergic antagonist that may be employed as an ophthalmic agent to manage glaucoma, or may be used as an antihypertensive agent in an oral dosage form.

9. d—Pioglitazone
    Pioglitazone is a thiazolidinedione agent employed in the management of diabetes mellitus. Nifedipine, propranolol, and procainamide are all used in the management of cardiovascular disorders.

10. c—Albuterol
    Albuterol is a beta agonist agent employed in the management of asthma.

11. a—Pravastatin
    Pravastatin is an HMG-CoA reductase inhibitor used in the management of hyperlipidemia. Fluconazole and nystatin are antifungal agents. Methylprednisolone is a corticosteroid.

12. a—Protease inhibitors
    Protease inhibitors are a category of antiretroviral agents.

13. c—Amlodipine
    Amlodipine is a calcium channel antagonist, while furosemide, hydrochlorothiazide, and triamterene are diuretic agents.

14. a—Pilocarpine
    Pilocarpine is a cholinergic agonist used to treat glaucoma. Ciprofloxacin is an antibiotic, naphazoline is an ophthalmic antiallergy agent, and atropine is employed as an ophthalmic diagnostic agent.

15. c—Macrolides
    Macrolides are a class of antibiotics.

16. c—Antiretrovirals
    Antiretroviral is the appropriate title for anti-HIV drugs.

17. c—Penicillamine
    Penicillamine is an agent employed against rheumatoid arthritis, and should not be confused with penicillin.

18. b—Permethrin
    Permethrin is used to manage infestations of lice.

19. d—Penicillin
    Penicillin (beta lactam antibiotic) is not an antiprotozoal medication.

20. b—Insulin glargine
    Insulin glargine (Lantus) is an ultra-long-acting insulin.

21. a—Mebendazole
    Mebendazole is an antihelmintic medication used in the management of worm infestations.

22. c—Alprazolam
    Diazepam and alprazolam are both benzodiazepines.

23. c—Enalapril
    Enalapril is used as an antihypertensive medication. Zolpidem is for insomnia, and sublingual nitroglycerin tablets are for angina.

24. c—Alendronate
    Alendronate (Fosamax) is a bisphosphonate used in the management of osteoporosis.

25. b—Anti-acne
    Isotretinoin (Accutane) is an anti-acne agent that is reserved for severe cystic acne.

Matching Answers

1. D	3. B	5. I	7. A	9. G
2. E	4. F	6. H	8. J	10. C

Apply Your Knowledge Answers

1. a. Antiarrhythmic
    b. Proton pump inhibitor/antiulcer agent
    c. Antidepressant/SSRI
    d. Cholinesterase inhibitor/anti-Alzheimer's agent
    e. HMG-CoA reductase inhibitor/cholesterol-lowering agent
    f. Insulin/antidiabetic agent
    g. Antihistamine/antiallergy
    h. Antiviral
    i. Oncologic/chemotherapeutic agent
    j. Thiazolidinedione/antidiabetic agent
2. Answers will vary.
3. Answers will vary.

Calculation Corner Answers

Solution

1. Which suspension will you use and why? Best choice is Amoxil 250 mg/5 mL suspension because less product is necessary to fill the prescription.
2. For the suspension you chose, calculate the milliliters required for each dose, total milliliters administered each day, and minimum quantity of suspension needed to prepare the prescription. If the student chose Amoxil 125 mg/5 mL:

125/5 = 200/X

125X = (200)(5)

$\quad$ X = (200)(5)/125

$\quad$ X = 8 mL per dose

Every 8 hours equals 3 doses per day, therefore

8 mL × 3 times a day = 24 mL/day

Ten days of treatment, therefore

24 mL/day × 10 days = 240 mL

If the student chose Amoxil 250 mg/5 mL:

250/5 = 200/X

250X = (200)(5)

$\quad$ X = (200)(5)/250

$\quad$ X = 4 mL per dose

Every 8 hours equals 3 doses per day, therefore

4 mL × 3 times a day = 12 mL/day

Ten days of treatment, therefore

12 mL/day × 10 days = 120 mL

Chapter 8 Lab

Multiple Choice Answers

1. d—Alternative medications
   Appropriate dose, active ingredient(s), and storage instructions are all found on the label of OTC medications.
2. a—Vitamin C
   Aspirin, acetaminophen, and ibuprofen are over-the-counter medications and are not marketed as dietary supplements.
3. c—Analgesics
   Analgesics are pain-relieving agents.
4. c—Antipyretics
   Antipyretics are fever-reducing agents.
5. b—Ibuprofen
   Ibuprofen is a nonsteroidal anti-inflammatory drug (NSAID).
6. c—Antihistamine
   Anesthetics are used to relieve irritation and decrease pain, antiemetics suppress nausea and vomiting, and analgesics relieve pain.
7. d—Patients with bone disorders
   Patients with diabetes, hypertension, or those being treated with antidepressants should always speak with their physician prior to taking over-the-counter oral decongestants. The sympathomimetic effects may exacerbate their conditions or interact with medications.
8. c—Antifungals
   Laxatives, antiemetics, and antacids are all categorized as gastrointestinal agents.
9. a—Fluoride
   Fluoride is incorporated into toothpastes to strengthen teeth.

10. d—Antibiotic
    Ophthalmic antiallergy, decongestant, and artificial tears agents are all available over-the-counter. Ophthalmic antibiotic agents are not available as nonprescription agents.
11. b—Suppresses cough
    Antitussive agents suppress cough.
12. d—Decreases nausea and vomiting
    An antiemetic agent suppresses nausea and vomiting.
13. b—Gastrointestinal
    Omeprazole is employed for relief of acid reflux and is used in the gastrointestinal system.
14. c—Hydrocortisone
    Clotrimazole, miconazole, and tolnaftate are all antifungal agents. Hydrocortisone is a corticosteroid.
15. d—Methylcellulose
    Methylcellulose is incorporated in gastrointestinal agents, while pseudoephedrine, diphenhydramine, and dextromethorphan are typically employed in cough and cold preparations.
16. b—Inactive ingredient(s)
    An excipient is the inactive ingredient(s) in the dosage form.
17. c—Child safety caps
    Tamper-evident packaging includes all of the following except child safety caps.
18. b—Aspirin
    Aspirin is associated with Reye's syndrome.
19. a—Salicylic acid
    Salicylic acid is an active ingredient used in wart removal agents.
20. b—Debrox
    Debrox may be used for earwax removal.
21. c—Pseudoephedrine
    Pseudoephedrine is an active ingredient in oral decongestants, not in nasal decongestant sprays.
22. d—Dementia
    There are home diagnostic kits available for pregnancy, ovulation, and illicit drugs.
23. c—Prilosec-OTC
    All of the choices are antihistamines except for Prilosec-OTC, which is a proton pump inhibitor.
24. d—Nicotine
    Nicotine is an active ingredient employed in smoking cessation products.
25. c—Patients should not see a physician if there is a foreign object in the eye.
    Patients *should* see a physician if there is a foreign object in the eye.

Matching Answers

1. B	2. C	3. A	4. E	5. D
1. C	2. A	3. D	4. E	5. B

Apply Your Knowledge Answers

1. The Food and Drug Administration (FDA) oversees the process of transitioning prescription-only preparations to over-the-counter available status. First, the drug sponsor submits data supporting the transition to the FDA. Then an OTC advisory committee and other consultants review the data. As a result of this review, a recommendation report is developed. If the advisory committee and consultants agree, a proposed monograph is developed and public comment is invited. The final monograph is prepared and reviewed. The last step in the process is the publication of the final monograph in the *Federal Register* and in the *Code of Federal Regulations*.

2. Answers will vary, but should include the following: Prilosec-OTC, TagametHB, Zantac75, Axid NR, Claritin, Motrin IB.

3. Answers will vary, but should include the following: refer the customer to the pharmacist, or indicate where the customer can find over-the-counter sleep aids in the store.

4. The patient should be referred to the pharmacist because it is likely that the preparations may affect her response to diabetes medications or, if it is a cough syrup, may contain sugar.

5. The patient should be informed that this is the same medication as the prescription he picked up, and he should be referred to the pharmacist or his physician prior to purchase.

Calculation Corner Answers

Solution

1. How many milliliters of Tylenol Infant's Drops should be given to Mrs. J.'s son in each dose?
   For the elixir:

   80 mg/2.5 mL = 160 mg/5 mL

   Mrs. J.'s son receives a total of 160 mg per dose as 1 tsp of the elixir is 5 mL.
   For the infant drops:

   80 mg/0.8 mL = 160 mg/1.6 mL

   Mrs. J.'s son should be given 1.6 mL of Tylenol Infant's Drops per dose.

Pharmacy Facts—Research Answers

1. Answers will vary, but should include: antiplatelet agents (for example: Ticlid (ticlopidine)), which can cause bleeding through duplicating aspirin's antiplatelet effects; anticoagulants (for example: Coumadin (warfarin)), which can cause bleeding; non-steroidal antiinflammatory agents (for example: Motrin (ibuprofen)), potentially increasing the risk of bleeding; and of course, other products containing aspirin (for example: Easprin (aspirin)).

2. Gingko biloba has increased the risk of bleeding when given with aspirin.

3. Answers may vary, but the following are examples.
   Anacin
   BC powder
   Excedrin Express Gels
   Alka Seltzer
   Bayer Aspirin

Chapter 9 Lab

Multiple Choice Answers

1. c—Standardization
   Standardization involves the consistency of components from batch to batch.

2. d—Homeopathy
   Homeopathy is based on the concept that toxins that may produce a given effect may be used in very small amounts to antagonize those symptoms.

3. b—Aromatherapy
   Aromatherapy is the inhalation of aromatic oils to produce a sense of well-being. Iridology is a diagnostic tool, while Rolfing and Shiatsu are types of massage therapy.

4. a—DSHEA
   The Dietary Supplement Health and Education Act of 1994 defines dietary supplements and regulations regarding marketing of the products.

5. b—Contamination
   Contamination is the presence of impurities in a product. Misbranding involves improper identification of the contents, while standardization involves consistency in contents of the same preparation.

6. c—Chiropractic medicine
   Chiropractic medicine involves the manipulation of the spine to restore or promote health and well-being.

7. d—Form of medicine originating in India that uses herbal preparations, dietary changes, exercises, and meditation to restore health and promote well-being
   Ayurvedic medicine originated in India and utilizes various methods to restore and promote health.

8. d—Western medicine
   Western medicine is not alternative therapy.

9. b—Dietary supplements
   All herbal agents marketed in the United States are considered dietary supplements because they have not undergone the rigorous clinical trials necessary for an agent to be marketed as a drug.

10. b—Iridology
    Iridology is used as a diagnostic tool, whereas chiropractic medicine, colonic therapy, and Chinese medicine are employed to manage or prevent maladies.
11. d—Date of manufacture
    The date of manufacture is not a labeling requirement for the dietary supplements.
12. d—Gingko and antiplatelet agents
    Inhibition of platelet aggregation and adhesion as a result of antiplatelet drug use combined with increased circulation as a result of gingko administration may result in increased risk of bleeding.
13. a—Ginseng and decongestants
    The combination of increased energy as a result of ginseng use with the sympathomimetic effects of the decongestants may cause nervousness and anxiety.
14. c—Increased sedation
    The combination of valerian, passionflower, or kava with benzodiazepines may result in increased sedation.
15. c—Adverse drug reaction
    An adverse drug reaction is a negative, nontherapeutic effect that occurs as a result of medication administration. A drug interaction involves two or more drugs, and a contraindication is a situation in which a medication should not be used.
16. b—Herbal preparations are safe because they are natural and nonsynthetic
    It is false that herbal preparations are safe because they are natural.
17. c—Comfrey
    Comfrey is considered to be unsafe in any amount.
18. d—Senna
    Senna exhibits cathartic (laxative) effects, not sedative effects.
19. d—Snakeroot
    Snakeroot is considered to be dangerous to humans.
20. b—Vitamin C
    Vitamin C is a water-soluble vitamin.
21. c—Arginine
    Arginine is an amino acid, not a mineral.
22. d—Folic acid
    Folic acid is administered to women of child-bearing age and pregnant women to reduce the risk of neural tube defects, like spina bifida.
23. d—Reduces triglycerides
    Omega-3 fatty acids are thought to reduce triglycerides and risk of heart disease.
24. d—Lactobacillus
    Lactobacillus is available in oral dosage forms and is incorporated into dairy products as a probiotic agent, which helps support the normal bacterial flora.

25. c—Soy
    Soy is marketed as an agent to help relieve the symptoms of menopause.

Matching Answers

1. J   2. A   3. F   4. H   5. C
6. B   7. I   8. D   9. G   10. E

Apply Your Knowledge Answers

1. Answers will vary, but should include the following: valerian, kava, passionflower vine.
2. Integrative medicine is the use of both traditional and alternative medical modalities to benefit the patient.
3. The over-the-counter medicine is evaluated by the FDA through clinical trials and is approved for use with specific indications. The labeling for dietary supplements cannot contain specific claims as they are not evaluated by the FDA to validate those claims.
4. Colonic therapy.
5. Chiropractic therapy involves adjustments of the spine to relieve pressure and/or pain.
6. Standardization.
7. Increased risk of bleeding.
8. Lactobacillus.
9. Glucosamine.
10. Melatonin.

Calculation Corner Answers

Solution

1. How much is this (2 gr of rose hips) in milligrams?
   1 gr = 60–65 mg
   2 gr = 2 (60)–2(65)
   The product contains 120–130 mg of rose hips.

Pharmacy Facts—Research Answers

Table 9-1

Agent	Claim
Acai	Appetite suppressant
Milk thistle	Liver protectant
Gingko biloba	Increases circulation, improves memory
Coenzyme Q10	Cardioprotective effects
Creatine	Enhances physical performance, builds lean body mass

Chapter 10 Lab
Multiple Choice Answers

1. d—Slower rate of therapeutic response
   Oral dosage forms take longer to demonstrate a therapeutic response because the drug must travel through the digestive system before it is absorbed into the body.
2. d—All of the above
   Intravenous medications bypass the digestive tract and therefore are not inactivated or destroyed like medications traveling through the digestive tract. Absorption is quicker because the drug is introduced directly into the bloodstream and therefore they reach the site of action sooner than an oral dosage form.
3. c—Intravenous
   Intradermal injections contain approximately 0.1 mL, intramuscular contain 2 to 5 mL, and subcutaneous injections contain less than 1 mL of fluid. Intravenous fluids may either be a small volume (less than 100 mL) or a large volume (greater than or equal to 100 mL) of fluid.
4. d—All of the above
   Creams, lotions, and ointments are administered topically.
5. d—All of the above
   A tablet contains an exact amount of medication and is easily identifiable due to the unique alphanumeric markings found on the tablet. Tablets are easy to administer because an individual does not need any special training to administer.
6. d—All of the above
   Binders, diluents, and disintegrants are components of tablets. Binders provide cohesiveness to the powdered material, diluents increase the size of the tablet to make it functional, and disintegrants aid in breaking up the tablet after it is administered.
7. d—All of the above
   Extended-release medications demonstrate regular absorption from the GI tract and are used to treat chronic conditions. They possess a good margin of safety that reduces the possibility of an overdose from occurring.
8. d—All of the above
   Capsules are easily administered because they do not require any special skills from the patient. Some capsules contain multiple active ingredients and are tasteless, resulting in improved patient compliance.
9. d—Used for potent drugs
   A transdermal dosage form cannot be used for potent medications due to the erratic rate of absorption of topical medications.
10. d—All of the above
    Suppositories may be administered rectally, placed inside the urethra, or inserted in the vagina.
11. d—Only select products are available for this route of administration
    A limited number of medications are available as a suppository due to their erratic rate of absorption into the body and the possibility they may be expelled from the body before the medication is absorbed.
12. d—All of the above
    All three states of matter (gas, liquid, and solid) can be dissolved into a solution.
13. d—All of the above
    Gargles, syrups, and suspensions may contain antiseptics, antibiotics, or anesthetics.
14. c—Protectant
    Alcohol is used to mask the unpleasant taste of active ingredients, flavoring is used to hide the unappealing taste of ingredients, and surfactants are used to aid in solubilizing flavoring agents in preparing a mouthwash. Protectants are not used in preparing mouthwashes.
15. b—Condensation of a sucrose solution through evaporation
    Syrups can be made by preparing a solution with the aid of heat, making a solution of the ingredients through agitation without the use of heat or adding sucrose to a prepared medicated or flavored liquid. Syrups cannot be made by evaporating a solution.
16. d—May not require the use of preservative in low concentrations (less than 10%)
    Elixirs may contain preservatives.
17. d—All of the above
    Tinctures need to be stored in a light-resistant and tightly closed container and must be stored away from heat.
18. c—Solution
    Solutions are not a disperse system because they contain one phase unlike aerosols, emulsions, and suspensions which have two phases.
19. d—All of the above
    Topical emulsions can either be O/W or W/O depending on the therapeutic agent being used, the desired effect of emulsion, and the physical condition of the skin.
20. d—All of the above
    Emulsifying agents should be colorless, odorless, and tasteless.
21. d—All of the above
    Air, bacteria, and light can affect the stability of an emulsion and therefore the storage of an emulsion is important.

22. a—Emulsion
    Lotions, magmas, and milks are types of suspensions; an emulsion is not a type of suspension.
23. b——Parenteral solutions
    One of the many ways parenteral solutions differ from other solution and dosage forms is that they must meet purity standards that are established in the *United States Pharmacopeia–National Formulary (USP–NF)*. These standards ensure their safety.
24. a—Parenteral solutions
    The use of coloring agents is prohibited by the *USP–NF*.
25. a—Large-volume parenteral
    Large-volume parenterals (LVPs) are a "ready-to-use system." Dextrose solutions can be used to replenish fluids and nutrients, sodium chloride can be to reload the body of fluids and electrolytes, and Lactated Ringer's injection can alkalinize the body and provide both fluids and electrolytes to the body.
26. d—All of the above
    Aerosols allow for lower dosages of a medication to be used; they provide a rapid onset of action and they are tamperproof.
27. d—All of the above
    Ophthalmic agents must examine the toxicity and isotonicity of a drug and the use of appropriate buffers and preservatives for the drug.
28. b—Poor patient compliance
    A medication error may occur if a pharmacy technician misinterprets a pharmacy abbreviation. Misinterpreting an abbreviation may result in the patient taking a wrong quantity of medication, taking the medication at the wrong time of day, or taking it by the incorrect route of administration.
29. a—In the intestine
    Enteric medications disintegrate in the intestine.
30. d—Under the tongue
    A sublingual tablet is placed under the tongue.

True/False Answers

1. False. Sublingual medications are placed under the tongue.
2. True.
3. False. Nitroglycerin can be administered sublingually, topically, transdermally, and through inhalation.
4. True.
5. True.
6. True.
7. False. Not all tablets can be chewed; only those indicated as chewable.
8. True.
9. True.
10. False. A diluent is an inert substance used to increase the size of a dosage form.
11. True.
12. False. There are many different types of extended-release products and each has a specific mechanism of action.
13. True.
14. True.
15. True.
16. True.
17. False. A solution consists of two phases: a solute and a solvent.
18. True.
19. True.
20. True.
21. False. Topical solutions may contain alcohol, but alcohol is not required for all topical solutions.
22. True.
23. True.
24. True.
25. True.
26. True.
27. False. Emulsions are extremely unstable.
28. True.
29. True.
30. True.
31. True.
32. True.
33. True.
34. False. Parenteral suspension must meet USP–NF criteria for purity.
35. True.

Abbreviations

aa—of each
ac—before meals
ad lib—freely
am—morning
bid—twice a day
caps—capsules
dtd—give of such doses
elix—elixir
emuls—emulsion
gtt(s)—drop(s)
h—hour
hs—at bedtime
kg—kilogram
lb—pound
mcg—microgram
mEq—milliequivalent
mg—milligram
mL—milliliter

non rep—do not repeat or do not refill
oint—ointment
pc—after meals
pm—afternoon
prn—as needed
qid—four times a day
rep—repeat
Rx—take this drug
Sig—write on label
sl—sublingual
sol—solution
stat—immediately
syr—syrup
tabs—tablets
tbsp—tablespoon
tid—three times a day
tsp—teaspoon
ung—ointment
vag—vaginal

Apply Your Knowledge Answers

1. Factors affecting the choice of ointment base would include the desired effect of the drug and the area of the body being treated.

2. Answers will vary based upon personal preference.
3. The final concentration would be ½ of the original concentration.
4. Many parents may not want an elixir to a child because of the alcohol content.
5. Shake Well because the medication is a suspension; Refrigerate because after amoxicillin is reconstituted it is stable for the greatest amount of time if it is refrigerated; Discard after10 days, because after amoxicillin is reconstituted, it is only good for 10 days.
6. Answers will vary based upon personal preference.
7. A suppository because both tablets and elixirs are an oral dosage forms and may be regurgitated from the body due to the nausea. Injectable dosage forms require an individual to have specific skills to perform an injection.
8. A suspension is more readily absorbed by the body than either a chewable tablet or capsule.
9. A patient would observe a faster onset of action and obtain a therapeutic level quicker.
10. Oral medications are easy to administer.

Practice Your Knowledge Answers

OTC Medication	Active Ingredients	Dosage Forms	Route of Administration
Afrin	oxymetazoline	Spray	Nasal
Aleve	naproxen sodium	Caplets, Gelcaps, Tablets	Oral
Benadryl	diphenhydramine	Tablet, capsule, caplet, elixir and syrup	Oral and topical
Caladryl	calamine and pramoxine	Suspension	Topical
Claritin	loratadine	Tablet	Oral
Contac	Acetaminophen, chlorpheniramine, dextromethorphan, phenlyephrine	Caplet	Oral
Cortaid	hydrocortisone	Cream and ointment	Topical
Debrox	carbamide peroxide	Drops	Ear
Delsym	dextromethorphan	Suspension	Oral
Epsom Salts	magnesium sulfate	Granule	Oral and topical
Hold	dextromethorphan	Lozenge	Oral
Imodium A-D	loperamide	Caplets and liquid	Oral
Lamisil AF	terbinafine	Cream, spray and powder	Topical
Medi-Plast	salicylic acid	patch	Topical
Metamucil	psyllium	Powder, capsules and wafers	Oral
Monistat 7	miconazole	Cream and suppository	Vaginal

(Continued)

OTC Medication	Active Ingredients	Dosage Forms	Route of Administration
Mylanta	aluminum hydroxide/ magnesium hydroxide	Suspension	Oral
Naphcon A	Naphazoline hydrochloride and pheniramine maleate	Solution	Ophthalmic
Ocean	normal saline	Spray	Nasal
Pepcid AC	famotidine	Tablets and Gelcaps	Oral
Pepto Bismol	bismuth subsalicylate	Liquid, chewable tablets and caplets	Oral
Preparation H	hydrocortisone	Cream, ointment, suppository	Rectal
Robitussin	guaifenesin	Syrup	Oral
Tylenol	acetaminophen	Tablets and caplets	Oral
Vitamin A	beta carotene	Capsule	Oral
Vitamin E	tocopherol	Capsule and oil	Oral and topical
Zantac	ranitidine	Tablet	Oral

Practice Your Knowledge Answers

Prescription Number	Error	Correction
1	Bactrim is not available as an elixir.	Bactrim is available as an oral suspension.
2	Rowasa is not available as a tablet.	Rowasa is either an enema or a suppository.
3	Otic	Should be ophthalmic-ear drops can't be placed in the eye.
4	Lipitor is not a sublingual tablet.	Lipitor is an oral tablet.
5	Coumadin is not available as intravenous drug.	Coumadin is an oral tablet.
6	Heparin is not available as a tablet.	Heparin is only available as an injectable solution.
7	Amoxicillin is not available as an elixir.	Amoxicillin is available as a liquid suspension.
8	Allegra D is not available as a capsule.	Allegra D is available as a tablet.
9	Xalantan is not available as a syrup.	Xalatan is a suspension.
10	Humulin N Insulin is not taken orally.	Humulin N Insulin is administered subcutaneously.

Calculation Corner Answers

Solution

1. How many grams of salicylic acid are required to prepare this compound? A 10% ointment means that 10 g of solute are contained in 100 g of the final product. One pound is equal to 454 g. The problem can be solved using a proportion:

$$\frac{10 \text{ g}}{100 \text{ g}} = \frac{X \text{ g}}{454 \text{ g}}$$

Cross-multiply:

$$(10 \text{ g})(454 \text{ g}) = (100 \text{ g})(X \text{ g})$$

Divide both sides of the equation by 100:

$$\frac{(10 \text{ g})(454 \text{ g})}{100} = \frac{(100 \text{ g})(X \text{ g})}{100}$$

$$X = 45.4 \text{ g}$$

You will need 45.4 g of salicylic acid to prepare this compound.

Pharmacy Facts—Research Answers

Table 10-1

Brand Name	Generic Name	Available Dosage Forms	Route of Administration For Each Dosage Form	Indication	List Five Side Effects
Advair	Fluticasone/salmeterol	Inhalation powder	Oral	Asthma	Answers will vary
Amoxil	amoxicillin	Capsules, tablets, chewable tablets and powder for oral suspension	Oral	Bacterial infection	Answers will vary
Biaxin	clarithromycin	Filmtab and granules	Oral	Bacterial infection	Answers will vary
Ciloxan	ciprofloxacin	Ointment and solution	Ophthalmic	Bacterial infection	Answers will vary
Cipro	ciprofloxacin	Tablets and oral suspension	Oral	Bacterial infection	Answers will vary
Demerol	meperidine	Oral solution and tablets	Oral	Analgesic	Answers will vary
Depakene	valproic acid	Liquid filled capsule and solution	Oral	Epilepsy Depression	Answers will vary
Dilantin	phenytoin	Extended oral capsule	Oral	Epilepsy	Answers will vary
Dovenex	calcipotriene	Ointment, cream and scalp solution	Topical	Psoriasis	Answers will vary
Go-Lytely	PEG	Oral solution	Oral	Bowel evacuant	Answers will vary
Haldol	haloperidol	Injection	Intramuscular	Psychosis	Answers will vary
Lidex	fluocinonide	Cream	Topical	Inflammation and itching associated with dermatoses	Answers will vary
Minocin	Minocycline	Suspension, capsule and injection	Oral and injectable	Acne	Answers will vary
Mycostatin	nystatin	Cream and powder	Topical	Fungal infections	Answers will vary
Proventil	albuterol	Inhalation aerosol	Oral	Asthma	Answers will vary
Reglan	metoclopromide	Tablet	Oral	Gastroesopheageal reflux	Answers will vary
Rowasa	mesalamine	Suspension enema	Rectal	Ulcerative colitis	Answers will vary
Terazol	terconazole	Cream and suppository	Vaginal	Fungal infection	Answers will vary
Thorazine	chlorpromazine	Tablet, spansule, syrup, ampules, multi-dose vial, and suppository	Oral, Intramuscular Rectal	Depression	Answers will vary
Zovirax	acyclovir	Capsule, tablet, suspension, ointment	Oral and topical	Herpes simplex	Answers will vary

Chapter 11 Lab

Multiple Choice Answers

1. d—Topical
   Products prepared using sterile compounding include intravenous admixture, irrigation solutions, and ophthalmic preparations.
2. b—Hyperalimentation
   Total parenteral nutrition is also known as hyper-alimentation.
3. a—USP <797>
   On January 1, 2004, the *United States Pharmacopeia* published USP<797>, a set of official and enforceable regulations governing sterile compounding.
4. b—Fever-producing agents
   Pyrogens are fever-producing agents.
5. c—Oral
   Sterile compounding is not required for medications that are administered orally.
6. d—All are potential sites for sterile compounding
7. d—Writing the medication order
   Writing medication orders is not a responsibility of the pharmacy technician.
8. d—All of the above
   The pharmacy is responsible for ensuring that sterile compounded products are free from contaminates, therapeutically appropriate, and properly labeled.
9. c—30 minutes
   The laminar flow hood should be turned on for at least 30 minutes before compounding begins.
10. b—IV additive machines
    Nondisposable equipment includes the laminar flow hood, compounding machines for TPN compounding, and other IV additive machines.
11. a—Horizontal
    The airflow in laminar flow hoods is either horizontal or vertical.
12. a—Parchment paper
    Parchment paper is disposed of after nonsterile compounding is completed.
13. c—Needles
    Personal protective equipment includes gloves, gowns, masks, eye protection, hair covers, and shoe covers.
14. b—Adding diluent to a powder for suspension or dissolution Reconstitution involves adding a diluent to a powder for suspension or dissolution.
15. a—Thorough and proper hand washing
    The pharmacy technician begins aseptic technique by thorough and proper hand washing.
16. b—Cleaned using 70% isopropyl alcohol
    The laminar flow hood must be cleaned using 70% isopropyl alcohol.

17. c—Filtered
    A filtered needle must be used when transferring liquid from an ampule to an IV bag.
18. b—Grinding particles
    Trituration involves grinding particles.
19. c—The HEPA filter
    The HEPA filter in the laminar flow hood should not be cleaned by the pharmacy technician.
20. d—An infection in the bloodstream
    Sepsis refers to an infection in the bloodstream.
21. b—Antibiotics
    TPN consists primarily of dextrose, amino acids, and lipids.
22. d—All of the above
    Sterile compounding of chemotherapeutic agents requires the use of a vertical laminar flow hood, proper aseptic technique, and proper hazardous waste disposal.
23. d—A closed front
    Gowns used while compounding sterile products should have a closed front.
24. c—Should be changed immediately
    Torn or damaged personal protective equipment should be changed immediately.
25. a—Speak or cough into the hood
    The pharmacy technician should not speak or cough in the hood.

True/False Answers

1. True.
2. False. The pharmacy technician is responsible for cleaning and maintaining the laminar flow hood and other pharmacy equipment and documenting the information.
3. True.
4. True.
5. False. Dispose of syringes and needles in a covered sharps container.
6. False. Compound one order at a time to avoid errors.
7. False. Do not attempt to remove or clean the HEPA filter in the laminar flow hood.
8. True.
9. True.
10. False. IV solutions should be checked for particulate matter before labeling.

Apply Your Knowledge Answers

1. USP <797>
2. TJC (formerly JCAHO)
3. Multiple vitamins, electrolytes, and insulin

4. Closed
5. Injury to the technician and glass particles in the medication

Calculation Corner Answers

Solution

1. What is the total amount (in grams) of ascorbic acid required to complete the order?

   120 mg × 20 = 2400 mg
   2400 mg ÷ 1000 = 2.4 g

   You will add 2.4 grams of ascorbic acid to complete the order.

2. How many milliliters of Gentamicin will you add to the IV bag?

   $\frac{60mg}{40mg} \times mL = 1.5mL$

   You will add 1.5 mL of Gentamicin to the IV bag.

Chapter 12 Lab

Multiple Choice Answers

1. d—All of the above
   A medication error is any preventable event that may cause or lead to incorrect medication use or patient harm while the medication is in the control of health professionals, health care product, procedures and systems, including prescribing; order communication; product labeling; packaging; nomenclature; compounding; dispensing; distribution; administration; education; monitoring and use.
2. b—Category B
   It is a Category B error because an error occurred but it was intercepted by the pharmacist before it reached the patient.
3. c—Category I
   This is a Category I error because the error did reach the patient and it may have caused the patient's death.
4. d—Anybody
   Anybody can commit a medication error regardless of age or experience.
5. d—All of the above are considered prescribing problems
   Prescribing errors include the following: the route of administration is not specified; patient allergies exist; incorrect strength of medication is indicated; incomplete medication name is on the prescription; quantity of medication and refills are not indicated; narcotics are refilled early; failure to provide a date

on the prescription; and incomplete directions on the prescription.
6. d—All of the above
   Making the pharmacy more ergonomically friendly, improving the lighting conditions, and reducing noise levels can actually help reduce medication errors.
7. c—Reduction of prescription problems and omissions errors
   Modifying current prescription pads to ensure consistency would eliminate many errors of omission by prescribers.
8. b—Omission errors
   MEDMARX has reported that 29% of medication errors are omission errors.
9. d—Performance deficit
   Performance deficit contributes to 38% of medication errors.
10. a—Human
    A knowledge-based error is an example of one caused by human factors.
11. d—All of the above
    Errors may result in injury or even death to a patient. As a result the individual responsible for the error may face legal consequences. A pharmacist has a legal responsibility to provide the patient with the best possible care. Failure to provide such care results in the pharmacist being charged with negligence.
12. d—None of the above
    There are no valid legal excuses for a prescription error.
13. d—All of the above
    Some of the goals established by the TJC include improving the accuracy of patient identification; improving the effectiveness of communication among caregivers; improving the safety of using high-alert medications; and improving the safety of infusion pumps.
14. d—All of the above
    The Institute for Safe Medication Practices (ISMP), The Joint Commission (TJC), and the United States Pharmacopeia (USP) conduct research and analyze data from this research. The data analysis examines trends on a monthly, quarterly, and yearly basis. These trends are cross-referenced by error category, error type, and cause of error.
15. b—TJC, formerly JCAHO
    The Joint Commission initiated the original list and the ISMP expanded the original list.
16. a—Informing the employee of the error
    The individual who committed the error should be informed of the error immediately. At that point, the organization should attempt to learn why and

how the error occurred and work to prevent the error from occurring again.

17. b—Informing the patient of the error
In the past, organizations have avoided telling the patient of the error for fear of potential lawsuits.

18. d—All of the above
Prescription errors can be caused by use of abbreviations; omissions on prescriptions; similar sounding and spelled medications; and medications that have been identified as "high-alert medications" that have resulted in a percentage of errors.

19. d—All of the above
The following categories of medications may cause harm to patients if taken incorrectly: adrenergic agonists, adrenergic antagonists, anesthetic agents, cardioplegic solutions, chemotherapeutic agents, dextrose, dialysis solutions, epidural or intrathecal medications, glycoprotein IIb/IIIa, hypoglycemic agents, inotropic agents, liposomal forms of medications, sedation agents, narcotics/opiates, neuromuscular blocking agents, radiocontrast agents, thrombolytic agents, and TPNs.

20. d—All of the above
The following agents can cause harm to a patient if taken incorrectly: amiodarone, colchicine injections, heparin, insulin, lidocaine, magnesium sulfate injection, methotrexate, nesiritide, nitroprusside, potassium chloride injection, potassium phosphate injection, sodium chloride injection, and warfarin.

21. c—Metric
The metric system is the approved system of measurement in the practice of pharmacy today. At one time both the apothecary and avoirdupois systems were used, but they contributed too many errors.

22. c—Contact the physician for clarification
If there is ever a question regarding a prescription, the prescriber should be contacted.

23. d—All of the above
Electronic prescribing eliminates illegible prescriptions, improves communication between the clinician and the patient, enhances communication throughout the prescribing chain, improves access to important reference and patient information, provides clinicians with cost information, and improves work efficiency.

24. d—All of the above
Proper staffing of the pharmacy during peak dispensing times, minimizing distractions such as phones ringing or loud music playing, ensuring the pharmacy is properly lighted, and providing ergonomic features to reduce an individual's fatigue can help reduce medication errors. Other ways to eliminate errors include arranging the inventory to differentiate the different medications and having a set of checks and balances in place during the prescription filling process.

25. c—Three times
A prescription should be read a MINIMUM of three times during the prescription-filling process.

26. d—All of the above
E-prescribing will improve patient safety and therefore improve the quality of the patient's care and allow the pharmacy to become more efficient in its day-to-day practices.

27. d—All of the above
Bar codes will be required to contain the NDC number, the lot (control/batch) number, and the expiration date. Bar codes should appear on all prescription and nonprescription medications regardless of the dosage form.

28. d—All of the above
It is important to discover the factual basis of a problem instead of the cause or nature of a problem. It is important to promptly record information regarding the situation and beneficial if a database can be maintained to identify commonalities of the situation to prevent the incident from occurring again.

29. a—FDA
The FDA oversees MedWatch, which serves both health care professionals and the public.

30. c—Vaccines
The Vaccine Adverse Event Reporting System (VAERS) is a cooperative program between the CDC and the FDA that provides post marketing surveillance of U.S.- licensed vaccines.

31. c—Hospitals
MEDMARX is a national, Internet-accessible database used by both hospitals and health care systems to track and trend adverse reactions and medication errors.

32. d—All of the above
Organizations using MEDMARX are able to improve patient safety and the standard of care within an institution; prevent medication errors and adverse drug reactions through protective measures to identify potential problems; eliminate high costs and risks associated with medication errors and adverse drug reactions; and provide insight into trends and best practices from a comprehensive national database.

33. d—All of the above
Medications Errors Reporting Program (MERP) is used by health care practitioners to identify errors caused by misinterpreting, miscalculating, and misadministering medications. It is also used to identify mediation orders that are difficult to interpret because they are handwritten; confusion over look-alike/sound-alike drugs; incorrect route of administration; and misuse of medical equipment.

34. d—All of the above
Patients can help reduce medication errors by using only one pharmacy, knowing the medication

they are taking, knowing their pharmacist, and maintaining a list of their medications.

35. d—All of the above

MEDMARX allows for the anonymous reporting of adverse drug events, captures information on actions taken and makes recommendations to avoid future adverse drug events, and provides for the completion of the TJC root cause analysis template and the FDA's MedWatch form.

True/False Answers

1. True.
2. True.
3. False. Bar codes do significantly reduce prescription errors.
4. False. There has been no "safe rate" for filling prescription regardless of the amount of experience an individual has.
5. False. Punishment is not an effective tool to prevent medication errors. It is more important to find the cause of errors and to correct them. Punishment may cause individuals not to report medication errors.
6. True.
7. True.
8. True.
9. True.
10. True.
11. True.
12. True.

Acronyms

APhA—American Pharmacists Association
CDC—Centers of Disease Control and Prevention
CQI—Continuous Quality Improvement
IOM—Institute of Medicine
ISMP—Institute for Safe Medication Practices
MERP—Medication Errors Reporting Program
NCVIA—National Childhood Vaccine Injury Act
PDCA—Plan-Do-Check-Act
TQM—Total Quality Management
VAERS—Vaccine Adverse Event Reporting System

Apply Your Knowledge Answers

1. Hydrochlorothiazide should be taken in the morning, not at bedtime.
2. The Controlled Substance Act limits the number of refills for Schedules III, IV, and V drugs to a maximum of 5 refills from the date the prescription is written.

3. Nitroglycerin is taken sublingually, not orally.
4. UD stands for "as directed"; however, "as directed" is not considered appropriate directions for the patient.
5. Demerol is not available as a 200-mg tablet.
6. Suppositories are not taken orally but rather inserted rectally in this situation.
7. One teaspoon of amoxicillin suspension is taken orally, not injected intravenously.
8. Prednisone is tapered downward, not built up.
9. Ibuprofen shouldn't be taken on an empty stomach because it may cause stomach irritation. Also, the dosage is excessive and above prescribed limits.
10. Ear drops should never be prescribed to be instilled into the eye. Also, the directions say to instill one drop in each eye as needed for ear infection.

Practice Your Knowledge Answers

Medication Prescribed	Confused Drug Names
Amaryl	Reminyl
Celebrex	Celexa, Cerebyx
Celexa	Zyprexa, Celebrex, Cerebyx
Clozaril	Colazal
Coumadin	Avandia
Cozaar	Zocor
Depakote	Depakote ER
Diovan	Dioval, Zyban, Darvon
Diprivan	Diflucan, Ditropan
Estratest	Estratest HS
Humulin	Novolin, Humalog
Inderal	Adderall
Kaletra	Keppra
Lanoxin	Levothyroxine
Lasix	Luvox
Lexapro	Loxitane
Lodine	Codeine, iodine
Maxzide	Microzide
Metformin	Metronidazole
Myleran	Alkeran, Leukeran
Numega	Neupogen
Pamelor	Panlor DC, Tambocor
Paxil	Doxil, Taxol, Plavix
Percocet	Darvocet, Procet
Prilosec	Prozac
Protonix	Lotronex, protamine
Reminyl	Robinul, Amaryl

(Continued)

Medication Prescribed	Confused Drug Names
Ritalin	Ritodrine
Roxanol	Roxicodone Intensol, Roxicet
Serafem	Serophene
Tegretol	Tegretol XR, Tequin, Trental
Tequin	Tegretol, Ticlid
Tobradex	Tobrex
Tylenol	Tylenol PM
Wellbutrin	Wellbutrin XL
Zebeta	Diabeta, Zetia
Zyprexa	Celexa, Reprexain, Zestril, Zyrtec
Zyrtec	Lipitor, Zantac, Zocor, Zyprexa, Zyrtec-D
Zyvox	Vioxx, Zovirax

Calculation Corner Answers

Solution

1. How long would it take to infuse 1 L of fluid? This is a rate problem and can be solved by using proportions. Convert liters to milliliters.

1 L = 1000 mL

Next set up a proportion:

$$\frac{100 \text{ mL}}{1 \text{ h}} = \frac{1000 \text{ mL}}{X \text{ h}}$$

Cross-multiply and divide:

$$\frac{100 \text{ mL} \times X \text{ h}}{100 \text{ mL}} = \frac{1 \text{ h} \times 1000 \text{ mL}}{100 \text{ mL}}$$

X = 10 h

It will take 10 hours to infuse 1 L of fluid.

Pharmacy Facts—Research Answers

Table 12-1

Brand Name	Generic Name	Strengths	Indications	Contraindications	Adverse Effects
Ancobon	flucytosine	250 and 500 mg capsules	Bacterial infections	None	Answers will vary
Combivir	lamivudine + zidovudine	Available in one 150/300mg	HIV	Patients with previously demonstrated hypersensitivity (anaphylaxis or Stevens-Johnson syndrome) to any of the ingredients	Answers will vary
Crixivan	indinavir	100,200 and 400 mg capsules	HIV	Patients taking amiodarone, cisapride, pimozide, alprazolam and triazolam.	Answers will vary
Diflucan	fluconazole	50, 100, 150 and 200 mg tablets; 10 or 40 mg/mL suspension; 2 mg/mL injection	Fungal infections	Hypersensitivity to flucanozole or other "azoles"	Answers will vary
Epivir	lamivudine	150 and 300 mg tablets; 10 mg/mL oral solution	HIV	Hypersensitivity (anaphylaxis) to lamivudine	Answers will vary
Flumadine	rimantadine	100 mg tablet; 50 mg/5 mL syrup	Flu	Patients showing hypersensitivity to drugs of adamantine class	Answers will vary
Fuzeon	enfuvirtide	90mg/vial	HIV	None	Answers will vary
Hivid	zalcitabine	0.375 and 0.75 mg tablet	HIV	None	Answers will vary
Invirase	saquinavir	200 mg capsules and 500 mg tablets	HIV	Patients with known hypersensitivity to saquinavar. amiodarone, quinidine, rifampin, cisapride, triazolam	Answers will vary

(Continued)

Table 12-1   (Continued)

Brand Name	Generic Name	Strengths	Indications	Contraindications	Adverse Effects
Lamisil	terbinafine	250 mg tablets	Fungal infections	None	Answers will vary
Lexiva	fosamprenavir	50mg/5 mL suspension and 700 mg tablets	HIV	Contraindicated with antiarrhythmics, antimycobacterials, ergot derivatives, GI motility agents, HMG CoA reductase inhibitors, neuroleptic agents , NNRTI's and sedatives.	Answers will vary
Loprox	ciclopirox	0.77% gel	Fungal infections	None	Answers will vary
Nizoral	ketoconazole	200 mg tablets	Fungal infections	Contraindicated with co administration of terbinafine or astemizole.	Answers will vary
Norvir	ritonavir	100 mg capsule and 80 mg/mL solution	HIV	Patients with known hypersensitivity to ritonavir; co administration with protease inhibitors, amiodarone, bepridil, flecainide, voriconazole, ergot derivatives, cisapride, lovastatin, simvastatin, and triazolam.	Answers will vary
Rescriptor	delaviridine	100 and 200 mg tablets	HIV	Patients with known hypersensitivity to any of its ingredients, astemizole, terbinafine, ergot derivatives, cisapride pimozide, alprazolam, triazolam	Answers will vary
Retrovir	zidovudine	100 mg capsule 10 mg/mL injectable solution 50 mg/5mL syrup 300 mg tablet	HIV	Patients who have had potentially life-threatening allergic reactions to any of its components.	Answers will vary
Sporanox	itraconazole	100 mg capsules	Fungal infection	Patients with ventricular dysfunction such as congestive heart failure, women who are pregnant or are considering pregnancy.	Answers will vary
Sustiva	efavirenz	50, 100, and 200 mg capsules 600 mg tablet	HIV	Antimigraine agents, benzodiazepines, calcium channel blockers, GI motility agents, neuroleptic agents and St John's Wort	Answers will vary
Symmetrel	amantidine	100 mg capsule 50 mg/mL syrup	Flu	None	Answers will vary
Terazol	terconazole	O,4 % and 0.8% cream; 80 mg suppositories	Vaginal yeast infection	None	Answers will vary
Trizivir	abacavir/ lamivudine/ zidovudine	One strength available (300mg/150 mg/300 mg) tablet	HIV	None	Answers will vary
Valtrex	valacyclovir	500 mg and 1 g tablets	Herpes simplex and CMV	Patients with known hypersensitivity to valcacylovir or acyclovir	Answers will vary

(Continued)

Table 12-1   (Continued)

Brand Name	Generic Name	Strengths	Indications	Contraindications	Adverse Effects
Videx	didanosine	Pediatric Powder for Oral Solution	HIV	Patients with known hypersensitivity to allopurinal, ribavirin	Answers will vary
Viracept	nelfinavir	250 and 625 mg tablet; 50 mg/g powder	HIV	Contraindicated with drugs that are dependent on CYP3A, amiodarone, quinidine, ergot derivatives, triazolam, pimozide	Answers will vary
Viramune	nevirapine	250 mg tablet; 50mg/5mL oral suspension	HIV	Patients with moderate or severe (Child Class B or C0 hepatic impairment.	Answers will vary
Viread	tenofovir	300 mg tablets	HIV	None	Answers will vary
Zerit	stavudine	10, 20, 30, and 40 mg capsules; 1 mg/mL oral solution,	HIV	None	Answers will vary
Zovirax	acyclovir	200 mg capsules, 5 % cream/ointment, powder for injection 500 and 1000mg/vial 50mg/mL injectable solution, 200mg/5mL suspension 400 and 800 mg tablets	Herpes simplex and CMV	Patients with known hypersensitivity to acyclovir or valacylovir.	Answers will vary

Chapter 13 Lab
Multiple Choice Answers

1. a—*Drug Facts and Comparisons*
   Drug Facts and Comparisons is updated monthly; *Red Book, Physicians' Desk Reference,* and the *United States Pharmacopeia* are updated yearly.
2. d—*United States Pharmacopeia*
   United States Pharmacopeia does not possess a drug identification section unlike *Drug Facts and Comparisons, Red Book,* or the *Physicians' Desk Reference.*
3. d—*United States Pharmacopeia Drug Information*
   United States Pharmacopeia Drug Information is published in three volumes. *Drug Facts and Comparisons, Red Book,* and the *Physicians' Desk Reference* are published as single volumes on a yearly basis.
4. b—*Red Book*
   Red Book is more valuable to community pharmacy practice because it contains reimbursement information, such as AWPs.
5. c—*The Injectable Drug Handbook*
   The Injectable Drug Handbook is more valuable to institutional pharmacies because of their use of injectable medications.

6. b—*Red Book*
   Red Book contains reimbursement information; the other three reference books do not.
7. d—*United States Pharmacopeia Drug Information*
   United States Pharmacopeia Drug Information contains both labeled and unlabeled uses of medication. *Red Book, Physicians' Desk Reference,* and *United States Pharmacopeia* contain information on labeled indications of a drug.
8. a—*American Hospital Formulary Service Drug Information*
   American Hospital Formulary Service Drug Information provides formulary information for hospitals. A formulary is an approved listing of medications used in both hospitals and managed-care organizations.
9. b—*Red Book*
   These are acronyms that are used in the reimbursement of medications to a pharmacy.
10. d—*Remington's Pharmaceutical Sciences*
    Remington's Pharmaceutical Sciences provides information regarding the practice of pharmacy in the United States. *American Drug Index* and *Goodman and Gillman's The Pharmaceutical Basis of Therapeutics* provides information regarding medications. *Martindale's Extra Pharmacopoeia* is a British version of *Remington's Pharmaceutical Sciences.*

11. d—All of the above
    Drug Topics, Pharmacy Times, and *U.S. Pharmacist* are a few of the many sources available to pharmacy technicians to obtain continuing education. Many sources can be found on the Internet and are free.

12. c—Nonproprietary
    A nonproprietary drug is another term for a generic drug. A proprietary name is synonym for a brand name or a trade name drug.

13. d—MEDMARX
    MEDMARX is used by hospitals to report medication errors allowing the information to be disseminated to other institutions to reduce the incidence of these errors from occurring again.

14. d—TOXLIT
    TOXLIT provides information regarding a drug's toxicity.

15. b—Chemical name
    A description of a medication includes a chemical description of the medication to include its chemical nomenclature and chemical formula.

16. d—Six
    There are six main sections and one miscellaneous section.

17. b—Hospital pharmacy
    The USP <797> focuses on maintaining aseptic conditions when preparing intravenous medications.

18. b—*USP Dictionary of USAN and International Drug Names*
    USP Dictionary of USAN and International Drug Names contains Japanese Accepted names.

19. d—P&T Committee
    The Pharmacy and Therapeutics (P&T) Committee consisting of physicians, pharmacists, and nurses develops a list of approved medications to be used in the institution.

20. c—*Ident-A-Drug*
    Ident-A-Drug provides a physical description of medication to include the dosage form, its color, and any alphanumeric markings on the medication.

21. c—*Neofax*
    Neofax contains pediatric information and is marketed to pediatric hospitals and institutions.

22. a—Epocrates
    Epocrates is software containing medication information and is downloaded to a PDA.

23. b—ACPE
    Accreditation Council for Pharmacy Education accredits pharmacy continuing education for both pharmacists and pharmacy technicians.

24. d—*U.S. Pharmacist*
    Each edition of *U.S. Pharmacist* is focused on a specific pharmacy related issue, such as a particular disease state.

25. b—MedlinePlus
    MedlinePlus works with the National Institutes of Health.

Apply Your Knowledge Answers

1. The usage of the medication.
2. Under what health conditions an individual should not use the medication.
3. The chemical description of a medication to include its generic name.
4. The mechanism of action of a medication; how the drug works in the body.
5. Warnings to the patient about taking the drug.
6. Side effects that have been reported, but it does not mean that an individual will experience them.
7. Method of treatment if an overdose should occur.
8. A listing of the various dosage forms available of the drug and its method of administration.
9. How the drug manufacturer supplies the medication in terms of packaging.
10. Clinical trials that have occurred.

Acronyms

ACPE—American College of Pharmacy Education
AERS—Adverse Event Reporting System
AWP—average wholesale price
CBER—Center for Biologics Evaluation and Research
CDER—Center for Drug Evaluation and Research
CEU—continuing education units
DP—direct price
NCPDP—National Council for Prescription Drug Programs
NDC—National Drug Code
NIH—National Institutes of Health
OBC—Orange Book Code
PDA—personal digital assistant
PDR—Physicians' Desk Reference
SRP—suggested Retail Price
USP–NF—United States Pharmacopeia–National Formulary
USPDI—United States Pharmacopeia Drug Information
VAERS—Vaccine Adverse Event Reporting System

Apply Your Knowledge Answers

1. I would use *Drug Facts and Comparisons* because it is marketed for the use in the pharmacy and it is updated on a monthly basis while the *Physician's Desk Reference* is marketed primarily to physicians and is updated on a yearly basis.
2. Yes, there is a 10% possibility that a person allergic to penicillin would be allergic to cephalosporins (i.e. Keflex). It would best to contact the physician and inform him or her of the situation and make the decision.

3. Yes, taking antibiotics while a female is using oral contraceptives may reduce the effectiveness of the oral contraceptives. The patient should be advised to use a secondary birth control method while taking the antibiotic.

4. No, a patient should not drink while taking Flagyl because the patient may experience severe adverse effects as a result of the interaction between Flagyl and alcohol.

5. Nexium is prescribed to treat stomach ulcers; taking naproxen simultaneously may aggravate these ulcers.

6. I would use *Remington's Pharmaceutical Sciences* because it provides general information regarding the practice of pharmacy and the steps in compounding various dosage forms.

7. *Injectable Drug Handbook*

8. Answers may vary but an individual can obtain continuing education units by attending seminars or by reading articles that have been approved by the ACPE.

9. It is awarded a "X" pregnancy code.

10. Ident-a-Drug provides and identification of drugs to include color and markings on the drug.

Practice Your Knowledge Answers

Drug Name and Strength	NDC Number	Drug Manufacturer	Recommended Daily Dose	Warnings
Humulin N Insulin 10 mL	na	Lilly	Dosage will vary based upon patient's need	Differs from animal source insulins and may require different dosage
Novolin 70/30 Insulin 10 mL	na	Novo Nordisk	Dosage will vary based upon patient's need.	Any changes in insulin should be made cautiously under medical supervision
Zithromax Z-pak	00069-3050-34	Pfizer	2 stat, 1 qd × 4 days	Contraindicated in patients sensitive to macrolides
Lipitor 10 mg 90 tablets	00071-0155-23	Pfizer	1 qd	Liver dysfunction; Category X pregnancy code
Serevent Inhaler	00173-0521-00	GlaxoSmithKline	One inhalation twice a day	Should not be used in acute situations
Depakote 500 mg 100 tablets	00074-6215-13	Abbott	750 mg daily in divided doses	Hepatotoxicity, Teratogenicity, Pancreatitis
Mysoline 250 mg 100 tablets	66490-0691-81	Valeant Pharmaceutical International	250 mg tid	Avoid abrupt withdrawal
Tessalon Perles	00456-0688-01	Forest Pharmaceuticals	100-200 mg po tid	Do not chew capsule
Diflucan 100 mg 100 tablets	00049-3240-41	Pfizer	100 mg po/IV qd	Caution with heart disease, renal impairment, hepatic impairment and elderly patients
Sinemet 25/250 100 tablets	00056-0654-68	Bristol–Myers-Squibb	1po tid-qid	Caution in patients having glaucoma, renal and hepatic impairment, asthma, endocrine disease or psychosis
Flonase Inhaler 14.2 mL	00173-0453-01	GlaxoSmithKline	2 sprays/nostril qd	Caution in patients with glaucoma, cataracts and adrenal suppression
Lidex cream 15g	99207-0511-13	Medicis	Apply bid-tid	Caution with skin infections
Coumadin 5 mg 100 tablets	00056-0172-70	BristolMyersSquibb	2-10 mg/qd	Has Black Box Warnings
Eskalith 300 mg 100 capsules	00007-4007-20	Noven Therapeutics	900-1200 mg/day	Has Black Box Warnings
Dilantin 100mg 1000 kapseals	00071-0369-32	Pfizer	300-400 mg qd	Caution if hypertensive, have cardiovascular disease, renal impairment, hepatic impairment, diabetes mellitus, and during pregnancy

(Continued)

Drug Name and Strength	NDC Number	Drug Manufacturer	Recommended Daily Dose	Warnings
Glucophage 850 mg 100 tablets	00087-6070-05	BristolMyersSquibb	850 mg bid	Has Black Box Warning
Proventil Inhaler 17 g	00085-1132-01	Schering-Plough	2 puffs q4-6 h prn	Caution if patient has arrhythmias, Hypokalemia, diabetes mellitus, seizure disorder, hyperthyroid or pregnant
Percodan 100 tablets	63481-0121-70	Endo	1 tab po q 6h	Aspirin triad. Caution if patient has bleeding disorder, respiratory depression or asthma
Efudex Cream	00187-3204-47	Valeant Pharmaceuticals	Apply twice a day for 2–4 weeks	Avoid excessive sun/UV light exposure
Micronase 5 mg 100 tablets	00009-0171-05	Pfizer	1.25 mg-20 mg po qd	Caution if pregnant, renal impairment, hepatic impairment, thyroid disease, adrenal insufficiency or elderly
Coreg 6.25 mg 100 tablets	00007-4140-20	GlaxoSmithKline	6.25 mg-25 mg bid	Caution if patient has bradycardia, heart failure, asthma, hepatic impairment. Avoid abrupt withdrawal.
Wellbutrin XL 150 mg 30 tablets	00173-0730-01	GlaxoSmithKline	300 mg po q am	Black Box Warning

Calculation Corner Answers

Solution

What is the total weight of this compound? The total weight of the compound can be calculated by adding the amount of each ingredient. In this situation, you would add the amount of each drug:

$$2 \text{ g} + 3 \text{ g} + 1 \text{ g} + 24 \text{ g} + 70 \text{ g} = 90 \text{ g}$$

The total weight of the compound is 90 g.

Pharmacy Facts—Research Answers

Table 13-1

Brand Name	Generic Name	Strengths	Dosage Forms	Indications	Contraindications	Adverse Effects
Accupril	quinapril	5, 10, 20 and 40 mg	Tablet	Hypertension	Pregnancy patients with a history of angioedema	Answers will vary
Aldomet	methyldopa	250 and 500 mg	Tablet	Hypertension	Patients with hepatic disease, liver disorders, taking MAO inhibitors	Answers will vary
Avapro	irbesartan	75 150 and 300 mg	Tablet	Hypertension	None	Answers will vary
Calan	verapamil	40, 80 120 mg	Tablet	Coronary artery disease	Patients with left ventricular dysfunction, Hypotension, 2nd or 3rd degree AV block, atrial flutter or fibrillation.	Answers will vary
Capoten	captopril	12.5, 25, 50 and 100 mg	Tablet	Hypertension	Pregnancy and angioedema	Answers will vary
Cardizem LA	diltiazem	120, 180, 240, 300, 360, and 420 mg tablets	Extended release tablet	Hypertension	Sick sinus syndrome, 2nd or 3rd degree AV block, hypotension, acute myocardial infarction	Answers will vary

(Continued)

Table 13-1 (Continued)

Brand Name	Generic Name	Strengths	Dosage Forms	Indications	Contraindications	Adverse Effects
Coreg	carvedilol	3.125, 6.25 12.5 and 25 mg	Tablet	Coronary artery disease	Bronchial asthma, 2nd or 3rd degree AV block, sick sinus syndrome, Bradycardia, hepatic impairment	Answers will vary
Corgard	nadolol	20, 40 and 80 mg	Tablet	Coronary artery disease	Bronchial asthma, sinus bradycardia, cardiogenic shock and cardiac failure	Answers will vary
Coumadin	warfarin	1, 2, 2 1/2 , 3, 4, 5, 6, 7 ½, 10 mg	Tablet and injection	Coronary artery disease	Pregnancy, bleeding disorders, patients suffering from alcoholism and psychosis	Answers will vary
Cozaar	losartan	25, 50 and 100 mg	Tablet	Hypertension	Pregnancy	Answers will vary
Crestor	rosuvastatin	None listed	Tablet	Hyperlipidemia	Pregnancy, liver disease and nursing mothers	Answers will vary
Diovan	valsartan	40, 80, 160 and 320 mg	Tablet	Hypertension	Pregnancy	Answers will vary
Hytrin	terazosin	1, 2, 5, 10 mg	Tablet	Hypertension	None	Answers will vary
Hyzaar	losartan/ hydrochloro-thiazide	50/12, 5, 100/12.5, 100/25 mg	Tablet	Hypertension	Pregnancy and patients with anuria or sensitive to sulfonamide drugs	Answers will vary
Inderal	propranolol	10, 20, 40, 60 and 80 mg	Tablets	Hypertension	Patients in cardiogenic shock, sinus Bradycardia, bronchial asthma	Answers will vary
Lanoxin	digoxin	0.125 and 0.25mg	Tablets	Coronary artery disease	Patients with ventricular fibrillation	Answers will vary
Lescol	fluvastatin	20 and 40 mg	Capsule and tablet	Hyperlipidemia	Liver disease	Answers will vary
Lipitor	atorvastatin	10, 20 40 and 80 mg	Tablet	Hyperlipidemia	Liver disease and pregnancy	Answers will vary
Lopid	gemfibrozil	600 mg	Tablet	Hyperlipidemia	Hepatic or severe renal dysfunction, gallbladder disease	Answers will vary
Lopressor	metoprolol	50 and 100 mg	Tablet and injection	Hypertension	Sinus Bradycardia, 2nd or 3rd degree heart block, cardiogenic shock, patients with a heart beat less than 45 beats/min	Answers will vary
Lotrel	Amlodipine/ benazepril	2.5/10, 5/10, 5/20, 5/40, 10/20 and 10/40 mg	Capsule	Hypertension	Angioedema	Answers will vary
Lovenox	enaparin	100mg/mL and 150mg/mL	Injection	DVT	Major bleeding, thrombocytopenia	Answers will vary
Mephyton	phytonadione	5 mg	Tablet	Coagulation disorders	None	Answers will vary
Mevacor	lovastatin	20 and 40 mg	Tablet	Hyperlipidemia	Liver disease	Answers will vary

(Continued)

Table 13-1   (Continued)

Brand Name	Generic Name	Strengths	Dosage Forms	Indications	Contraindications	Adverse Effects
Minipress	prazosin	1 mg	Capsule	Hypertension	Sensitivity to quinazolines	Answers will vary
Nor pace	disopyramide	100 and 150 mg	Capsule	Coronary artery disease	Cardiogenic shock, pre-existing 2nd or 3rd degree AV block	Answers will vary
Norvasc	amlidopine	2.5, 5 and 10 mg	Tablet	Hypertension	None	Answers will vary
Persantine	dypridamole	25, 50 and 75 mg	Tablet	Coronary artery disease	None	Answers will vary
Plavix	clopidogrel	75 and 300 mg	Tablet	Coronary artery disease	Pathological bleeding due to peptic ulcer or intracranial hemorrhage	Answers will vary
Pravachol	pravastatin	10, 20, 40 and 80 mg	Tablet	Hyperlipidemia	Liver disease	Answers will vary
Procardia	nifedipine	10 mg	Capsule	Coronary artery disease	None	Answers will vary
Tenormin	atenolol	25, 50 and 100 mg	Tablet	Hypertension	Sinus Bradycardia, cardiogenic shock and cardiac failure	Answers will vary
Trental	pentoxifylline	400 mg	Tablet	Intermittent claudication with patients with chronic occlusive arterial disease	Cerebral or retinal hemorrhage	Answers will vary
Vaseretic	enalapril/ hydrochloro-thiazide	10/25 mg	Tablet	Hypertension	Angioedema and pregnancy	Answers will vary
Vasotec	enalapril	2.5, 5, 10 and 20 mg	Tablet	Hypertension	Angioedema and pregnancy	Answers will vary
Zestril	lisinopril	2.5, 5, 10, 20, 30 and 40 mg	Tablet	Coronary artery disease	Pregnancy	Answers will vary
Zetia	ezetimibe	10 mg	Tablet	Hyperlipidemia	Liver disease, pregnancy, nursing mothers	Answers will vary
Zocor	simvastatin	5, 10, 20, 40 and 80 mg	Tablet	Hyperlipidemia	Liver disease, pregnancy, nursing mothers	Answers will vary

Chapter 14 Lab

Multiple Choice Answers

1. a—Chain pharmacy
   CVS and Walgreens are both chain pharmacies.
2. d—State board of pharmacy
   The state board of pharmacy is responsible for the practice of pharmacy within the state and therefore issues a permit to the pharmacy allowing it to purchase and dispense medications.
3. d—All of the above
   All pharmacy laws must be followed by a pharmacy.
4. a—DAW 0
   DAW 0 indicates the prescriber has approved the use of a generic drug to be dispensed.
5. b—Signa
   The signa are the directions to the patient. These directions inform the patient when to take the medication, how much to take at a specific time, and the route of administration.
6. b—DAW 1
   DAW 1 because the physician has written on the prescription "Brand Name Medically Necessary."
7. c—FS3692464
   The first letter must be an "A," "B," "F," or "M." The second letter is the first letter of the prescriber's

last name. The set of numbers follows a numerical formula where you add the first, third, and fifth numbers of the series. Next you add the second, fourth, and sixth numbers of the series and multiply the sum of this series by two. Then add the sum of the first series of numbers to the product of the second series of numbers. The number in the one's column after adding two series of numbers should be the seventh number.
8. d—All of the above
   Auxiliary labels provide additional information to the patient regarding taking the medication, storing the medication, or experiencing potential adverse effects. All three of them are auxiliary labels.
9. a—Co-pay
   A co-pay is the amount of money an individual needs to pay. A deductible refers to the amount of money that must be paid before the insurance will reimburse. Fee for service refers to a component of the reimbursement formula. The premium refers to how much an individual must pay for the coverage of the plan.
10. c—DAW 2
    DAW 2 indicates a prescriber has approved the dispensing of a generic medication but the patient is requesting the brand-name medication be dispensed.
11. d—All of the above
    A retail pharmacy must follow all local laws, state laws, and federal laws. If two laws conflict, the pharmacy must follow the more stringent of the two laws.
12. a—Counsel patients
    At this time, pharmacy technicians are not permitted to counsel a patient about their medication.
13. d—Subscription
    The subscription indicates whether a refill has been approved by the prescriber and how many refills have been approved.
14. a—7 days
    Divide the number of tablets dispensed by the maximum number of tablets taken in one day: 60 tablets/8 tablets per day is equal to a 7 ½-day supply of medication.
    Hint: When dealing with a partial day always round down.
15. b—6789
    The middle set of numbers indicates the drug product.

True/False Answers

1. True.
2. False. The signa bid are the directions to the patient to take this drug twice a day

3. False. The Rx symbol informs the pharmacist what medication is to be dispensed. The sig(na) are directions to the patient on how to take the medication.
4. True.
5. True.
6. True.
7. True.
8. False. A pharmacy technician can accept a faxed prescription from a physician's office; he or she cannot take a new phoned-in prescription from the doctor's office.
9. True.
10. False. A faxed prescription is not an example of e-prescribing. E-prescribing is when a physician's office sends a prescription electronically from the physician's computer directly to the pharmacy computer through a secure system.

Matching Answers

1. H	5. D	9. E	13. G	17. O
2. A	6. J	10. F	14. T	18. P
3. M	7. B	11. L	15. S	19. Q
4. K	8. I	12. C	16. N	20. R

Acronyms

CMS—Centers for Medicare and Medicaid Services
CPOE—computerized physician order entry
DAW—dispense as written
DEA—Drug Enforcement Administration
DUE—Drug Utilization Evaluation
HIPAA—Health Insurance Portability and Accountability Act
HMO—health maintenance organization
IPA—independent practice association
MAC—maximum allowable cost
NDC—National Drug Code
NPI—National Provider Identifier
OBRA—Omnibus Reconciliation Act
OTC—over-the-counter
PBM—prescription benefit manager
PPO—preferred provider organization

Apply Your Knowledge Answers

1. Contact the physician, explain the situation and ask the physician to change the prescription to a medication that is covered under the insurance plan.
2. Explain to the patient that their prescription plan pays for a 30-day supply of medication only at a community pharmacy and they would need to return to the pharmacy on a monthly basis. You may remind the patient that they have a mail order option with their prescription plan that allows them to obtain a 90-day supply.

3. Explain to the patient that although their physician has informed them they will need to take the medication the remainder of their lives, state law allows a non-controlled prescription to be valid up to one year from the date it is written.

4. Inform the pharmacist of the situation; they will investigate and make a decision on whether to fill the prescription or contact the physician.

5. Answers will vary based upon the student's environment and their personal experiences with a chain pharmacy, independent pharmacy, mass merchandiser or grocery store.

6. Advantages: Convenience because the customer does not need to park their car and walk into the pharmacy to drop off or pick up their prescription. Disadvantage: They may not be able to make non-prescription purchases from the drive-thru window.

7. The pharmacy technician can make sure they have the patient's most current prescription drug card and the patient's information is correct. Secondly, the pharmacy technician can be familiar with various prescription drug plans as far as locating the information on the card and entering it into the computer system.

8. Collecting accurate information from the patient may reduce possible contraindications and eliminate adverse drug interactions.

9. Advantages; Saves time in prescription processing and eliminate unnecessary charges when resubmitting a prescription drug claim.
   Disadvantages: The prescription benefit managers would need to come to agreement on the requirements and it may be extremely expensive in both terms of time and money to implement and therefore may affect patient care.

10. No, many pharmacy technicians do not have a broad enough knowledge base to be able to answer all questions posed by a customer.

Practice Your Knowledge Answers

(Answers will vary.)

Drug Classification	OTC Product	Active Ingredients	Dosage Form	Drug Interactions	Warnings
Analgesic					
Antidarrheal Agent					
Antifungal agent					
Antiseptic agent					
Carminative					
Contact lens agent					
Cough suppressant					
Dietary supplement					
Disinfectant					
Expectorant					
First aid agent					
Laxative					
Local anesthetic					
Non-steroidal; anti-inflammatory agent					
Nutritional supplement					
Stool Softener					
Topical analgesic					
Topical antibiotic					
Vitamin					

Calculation Corner Answers

Solution

How many days will the prescription last the patient?

$$\text{Day's supply} = \frac{\text{Quantity dispensed}}{\text{Quantity taken each day}}$$

One day's supply is 40 capsules. If four capsules are taken each day, then the prescription will last the patient 10 days.

Pharmacy Facts—Research Answers

Table 14-1

Brand Name	Generic Name	Indication	List Five Side Effects	Is This Medication a Controlled Substance?
Advair Diskus	fluticasone/salmeterol	Asthma	Answers will vary	No
Ambien	zolpidem	Insomnia	Answers will vary	Yes
Amoxil	amoxicillin	Bacterial infection	Answers will vary	No
Coumadin	warfarin	Blood thinner	Answers will vary	No
Fosamax	alendronate	Osteoporosis	Answers will vary	No
Lasix	furosemide	Diuretic	Answers will vary	No
Lexapro	escitalopram	Depression	Answers will vary	No
Lipitor	atorvastatin	Hyperlipidemia	Answers will vary	No
Nexium	esomeprazole	GERD	Answers will vary	No
Norvasc	amlodipine	Hypertension	Answers will vary	No
Prevacid	Lansoprazole	GERD	Answers will vary	No
Protonix	pantoprazole	GERD	Answers will vary	No
Singulair	montelukast	Asthma	Answers will vary	No
Synthroid	levothyroxine	Hypothyroidism	Answers will vary	No
Toprol XL	metoprolol	Hypertension	Answers will vary	No
Vicodin	hydrocodone/acetaminophen	Analgesic	Answers will vary	Yes
Zestril	Lisinopril	Coronary artery disease	Answers will vary	No
Zithromax	azithromycin	Bacterial infection	Answers will vary	No
Zoloft	sertraline	Depression	Answers will vary	No
Zyrtec	cetirizine	Respiratory allergy	Answers will vary	No

Chapter 15 Lab

Multiple Choice Answers

1. d—PTCB
   PTCB stands for Pharmacy Technician Certification Board which is the organization that certifies pharmacy technicians and has no jurisdiction over inpatient pharmacies. TJC has jurisdiction over inpatient pharmacies.
2. a—CPOE
   CPOE stands for computerized physician order entry.
3. b—Unit-dose
   A single packaged dose of medication is a unit-dose.
4. b—Formulary
   A formulary is a list of medications available for use in a facility.
5. d—All of the above are acceptable
   Verbal, written, and electronic are all acceptable forms of medication orders.
6. b—STAT order
   A STAT order is used to indicate that the medication is needed immediately.

7. b—Pharmacy and Therapeutics Committee
   The Pharmacy and Therapeutics Committee is responsible for establishing and updating the hospital formulary.
8. c—TJC, formerly JCAHO
   The Joint Commission (TJC) accredits hospitals.
9. d—Substituting a drug from the same therapeutic class
   Therapeutic substitution involves substituting a drug from the same therapeutic class.
10. c—Protocol
    A protocol is a set of guidelines and standards governing procedures or medication administration in a facility.
11. c—Daily
    According to the TJC's (formerly JCAHO's) "Do Not Use" list, "daily" should be written to indicate that a medication is to be administered once a day.
12. d—Social Security number
    The patient's Social Security number is not included in his or her medication profile.

13. b—Prn order
    A prn order is used to indicate that a patient is to receive medication as needed.
14. a—Centralized model
    A centralized model pharmacy is an inpatient facility that has a single pharmacy that serves all areas of the medical center.
15. a—Medication administration
    Medication administration is not a responsibility of the inpatient pharmacy technician.
16. a—The pharmacy technician should use hypoallergenic gloves
    If a pharmacy technician is allergic to latex gloves the pharmacy technician should use hypoallergenic gloves.
17. c—Right technician
    The five rights of medication administration are right patient, right drug, right dose, right time, and right route.
18. d—Insurance coverage
    The patients' insurance coverage is not included on the medication label.
19. b—Decentralized system
    A pharmacy system involving multiple pharmacies serving various areas in a facility is called a decentralized system.
20. b—USP <797>
    USP <797> is a set of enforceable regulations governing compounding.
21. a—Has more than 500 patient beds
    Community hospitals have 25 to 100 beds.
22. c—FDA
    The FDA has no jurisdiction over inpatient facility standards.
23. c—Procedures
    Procedures are the steps or methods by which the regulations of an inpatient facility are carried out.
24. a—Be included before the decimal, as in 0.X mg
    According to TJC's "Do Not Use" list, a zero should be included before the decimal as in 0.X mg.
25. b—OSHA
    OSHA enforces standards relating to the safety of the workforce.

Matching Answers

1. D   2. C   3. B   4. A   5. E

Apply Your Knowledge Answers

1. Answers will vary, but should include the following: signs are posted; access is limited; eating, drinking, and/or smoking are prohibited in the area.

2. Inventory management, sterile compounding, medication order processing, medication distribution, data entry.
3. Automation.
4. Formulary.
5. Unit-dose medications.
6. The pharmacist is ultimately responsible.
7. Answers will vary, but should include the following: medication delivery, sterile compounding, stocking automated systems, inventory management, floor stock inspection, medication order processing.
8. Answers will vary, but should include the following: OSHA is the Occupational Safety and Health Administration, which ensures the safety and health of the workforce by setting and enforcing standards; providing training, outreach, and education; establishing partnerships; and encouraging continual improvement in workplace safety and health. The purpose of OSHA is to prevent work-related injuries, illnesses, and deaths.
9. Answers will vary, but should include the following: assisting in the training of pharmacy technician students and new hires, serving on ad hoc committees, preparing investigational drugs, providing training to others regarding the use of automated equipment.
10. Right patient, right drug, right dose, right time, and right route.

Calculation Corner Answers

Solution

1. How many grams of dextrose are contained in 100 mL D5W?

   1. 5% = 5/100
   5/100 = X g/100 mL
   5/100 = 5 g/100 mL

   5 g of dextrose are contained in 100 mL D5W.

2. How many grams of dextrose are contained in 500 mL D5W?

   2. 5% = 5/100
   5/100 = X g/500 mL
   (500) 5/100 = X
   X = 25 g/500 mL

   25 g of dextrose are contained in 500 mL D5W. There is an alternate solution to computing question 2. Using the solution to question 1, you know that there are 5 g in 100 mL, so 500 mL is 5 times the volume of 100 mL and, at the same concentration, contains 5 times the dextrose:

   $5 \times 5 \text{ g} = 25 \text{ g}$

Pharmacy Facts—Research Answers

Table 15-1

Brand Name	Generic Name	Therapeutic Classification	Dosage Forms
Versed	midazolam	benzodiazepine	injection
Hep-lock	heparin	anticoagulant	injection
Reglan	metoclopromide	GI motility agent	tablet, injection
Rocephin	ceftriaxone	cephalosporin antibiotic	injection
Kytril	granisetron	antiemetic	tablet, oral solution
Synthroid	levothyroxine	thyroid supplement	tablet, injection
Vasotec	enalapril	ACE inhibitor	tablet, injection
Lopressor	metoprolol	beta blocker	tablet, injection
Vancocin	vancomycin	antibiotic	capsules, injection

Chapter 16 Lab

Multiple Choice Answers

1. d—All of the above
   A long-term care facility is one that provides services to a patient who needs to be hospitalized for more than 30 days. Chronic disease hospitals, hospice care, and nursing homes are all examples of long-term care facilities.
2. d—All of the above
   Long-term care facilities provide health care, personal care, and social services for their residents.
3. a—Adjudication
   Adjudication is the process by which a pharmacy bills a prescription to a third-party provider or PBM.
4. d—Managed-care pharmacy
   Managed-care pharmacies perform audits to ensure the proper billing of prescriptions to the PBM.
5. d—Mail-order pharmacy
   A mail-order pharmacies would not prepare a TPN because they provide medications for chronic conditions. Unlike medications for chronic conditions, TPNs have specific storage and beyond-use dating requirements.
6. b—Long-term pharmacy
   Long-term care pharmacies are required to dispense unit-dose medications and therefore pharmacy technicians may be required to repackage medications from a bulk container.
7. d—Nuclear pharmacy
   Only nuclear pharmacies prepare and dispense radionucleotides.
8. d—All of the above
   Epidural, intravenous, and subcutaneous medications are all injected into the body through the use of a needle.
9. d—All of the above
   All pharmacies regardless of their setting are required to maintain a library of reference material applicable to their practice.
10. d—All of the above
    Mail-order pharmacies provide a cost savings to patients because the patients are able to receive a larger quantity (90-day supply instead of a 30-day supply from a retail pharmacy) and the pharmacies are capable of maintaining a larger inventory of medications than retail pharmacies.
11. d—All of the above
    The home infusion market is expanding because of the increased number of people who are living longer that may require this service. The quality of vascular lines is improving, which allows many individuals to receive home infusions in their homes at a much lower cost than receiving them in the hospital. Both physicians and insurance providers encourage patients to receive infusions in their homes if the patients have the proper resources.
12. b—Long-term care pharmacy
    Long-term care pharmacies allow patients to return unused medication to the pharmacy because the medication is in unit-dose packaging. This type of packaging allows pharmacists to determine if the medication has been tampered with.
13. b—Prepare sterile medication orders
    A pharmacy technician would prepare sterile medications to be infused in the patient.
14. c—PBM
    A prescription benefit manager designs a prescription drug plan based on the client's criteria, and then administers and manages the

plan. HMOs, IPAs, and PPOs are types of managed-care plans.

15. c—TRICARE
TRICARE is a federal third-party provider that administers health benefits to the dependents of military personnel.

16. d—Part D
Medicare Part D allows Medicare recipients to enroll in this third- party prescription plan and obtain their medications at a retail pharmacy using a third-party drug card.

17. d—All of the above
PBMs control costs by limiting the day's supply (normally 30) of a medication a patient may receive at a single time at a retail pharmacy. They do not cover all medications by developing "exception lists" of drugs not covered under a plan or possibly implementing a formulary. Finally, online adjudication is required of participating pharmacies and as a result helps control administrative costs.

18. d—All of the above
During Drug Utilization Evaluation (formerly known as Drug Utilization Review) the pharmacist is notified of all possible contraindications, drug interactions, and under- or overdosing based on the information collected from the patient and contained in the patient profile.

19. d—All of the above
Managed care provides high-quality medications to a patient at a reasonable cost at a pharmacy that is convenient to the patient.

20. d—All of the above
Analgesics, antibiotics, and TPNs can be made for infusion into a patient at a home infusion pharmacy.

21. d—Pharmaceutical company
A pharmaceutical company does not perform a Drug Utilization Evaluation because it is not dispensing medications to a patient but rather dispensing information and selling medications to both physicians and pharmacists.

22. d—All of the above
Some of the many rejection codes that a pharmacist or pharmacy technician may experience during the online adjudication process include "drug not covered," "patient not covered," and "refill too soon."

23. d—All of the above
OBRA-87 requires that all medications dispensed be in unit-dose packaging. Unused controlled substances cannot be returned to a pharmacy from a long-term care facility because the facility does not possess a DEA number. A system must be in place to track the reissuing of unit-dose medications in case of a possible medication recall.

24. c—Prepare radionucleotides
Pharmacy technicians would not prepare radionucleotides in a long-term care pharmacy. Radionucleotides are prepared at nuclear pharmacies.

25. a—Certificate of Medical Necessity and Plan of Treatment
Physicians must complete a Certificate of Medical Necessity and Plan of Treatment prior to a home infusion pharmacy preparing and dispensing injectable medications to be administered in a patient's home.

True/False Answers

1. False. All prescription medications require a prescription from a licensed prescriber before they can be dispensed to a patient even in an emergency.

2. False. OBRA-90 required that Drug Utilization Evaluation be performed on prescription orders regardless of the pharmacy setting.

3. True.

4. False. VIPPS stands for Verified Internet Pharmacy Practice Site and indicates the pharmacy is a legitimate pharmacy and meets specific guidelines and not a "rogue" pharmacy site.

5. False. Pharmacy technicians may prepare medications for home infusion patients but do not administer the medications to the patients.

6. True.

7. True.

8. False. A pharmaceutical sales or detail person provides drug information to both pharmacies and physicians.

9. False. Pharmacists working in a mail-order pharmacy are required to counsel any patients who may have questions about their medications. Every patient receives printed information about the medication and a pharmacist is available 24 hours a day to answer any patient questions.

10. False. In addition to being a certified pharmacy technician, they must obtain additional training regarding nuclear medicine. Additional credentials are often required by state boards of pharmacy.

11. False. Radiation is not used in home infusion pharmacy but rather is used in nuclear pharmacy.

12. True.

13. False. Radiopharmaceuticals are prepared in a nuclear pharmacy, not a home infusion pharmacy.

14. False. Often a long-term care pharmacy is not found in a long-term care facility. A long-term care pharmacy may either be an open or closed shop pharmacy. An open shop pharmacy provides medications for both regular patients and residents of a long-term care facility. A closed shop pharmacy

provides medications only to residents of a long-term care facility.

15. True.

Acronyms

ASHP—American Society of Health-System Pharmacists

CDC—Centers for Disease Control and Prevention

DHS—Department of Health and Human Services

DME—durable medical equipment

DUE—Drug Utilization Evaluation

HMO—health maintenance organization

IHS—Indian Health Services

IPA—independent practice association

IV—intravenous

MCO—managed-care organization

NABP—National Association of Boards of Pharmacy

NIH—National Institutes of Health

P&T—Pharmacy and Therapeutics

PBM—prescription benefit manager

PPO—preferred provider organization

TJC—The Joint Commission

VIPPS—Verified Internet Pharmacy Practice Site

Apply Your Knowledge Answers

1. I would dispense a thirty day supply of medication to the patient and change the number of refills permitted on the prescription. I would explain to them that their managed care organization will only pay the pharmacy for a thirty day supply of medication and if they have any additional questions refer them to their employee benefits department or third party provider.

2. Answers will vary depending on the interests of the student and possibly the career opportunities in their community.

3. A pharmacy technician working in a home infusion pharmacy needs to have strong math skills and USP<797>. In addition, they need to have excellent skills in preparing intravenous and other injectable preparations.

4. Long-term care facilities will vary depending on the community. Omnicare (formerly NeighborCare) is a long-term care pharmacy provider.

5. I believe interpersonal skills are more important because an individual must communicate effectively with other health care professionals when providing information to them.

6. Answers will vary but they may include Nitroglycerin, Glucagon for Injection, Heparin, Coumadin, Lovenex, Epi-Pen and Dilantin, Medications found in a "crash cart" are used in life threatening situations.

7. Pharmacist oversee the work of pharmacy technicians in preparing home infusion medications; pharmacy technicians to assist the pharmacist in preparing home infusion medications; inventory specialists are needed to ensure that appropriate levels drugs and various vehicles such as D5W, D10W, and NS are maintained; billing specialists to ensure proper reimbursement for intravenous medications and drivers to make sure the preparations are delivered to the patients.

8. Managed care provides the patient with cost savings with their medications and the patient has access to a pharmacist 24/7/365 to answer questions. Some of the disadvantages include formulary, day's supply and refill restrictions. Many individuals lack are unable to establish a rapport with the pharmacist.

9. The patient benefits from a fixed co-payment if the medication is expensive and from a % co-payment if the prescription is extremely inexpensive. There is no advantage for the pharmacy for either system because their reimbursement is described in their contract with the third party prescription provider.

10. The PBM benefits from a drug formulary because they are able to determine which medications will be covered under the prescription and will maximize their profitability.

Calculation Corner Answers

Solution

1. How many units of ampicillin will the patient receive after 15 minutes? This problem can be solved using proportions.

   Step 1: Set up a proportion:

   $$\frac{1.25 \text{ million units}}{30 \text{ minutes}} = \frac{X \text{ units}}{15 \text{ minutes}}$$

   Step 2: Cross-multiply:

   $$(1.25 \text{ million units})(15 \text{ minutes}) = (30 \text{ minutes})(X \text{ units})$$

   Step 3: Divide both sides of the equation by 30 minutes:

   $$\frac{(1.25 \text{ million units})(15 \text{ minutes})}{30 \text{ minutes}} = \frac{(X \text{ units})}{30 \text{ minutes}}$$

   Step 4:

   $$X = 625{,}000 \text{ units}$$

   The patient will receive 625,000 units of ampicillin after 15 minutes.

Pharmacy Facts—Research Answers

Table 16-1

Brand Name	Generic Name	Drug Classification	Dosage Forms	List Two Indications Of the Medications	List Three Adverse Effects Of the Medication
Advair	fluticasone/ salmeterol	beta adrenergic/ corticosteroid combination	Spray powder	Asthma	Answers will vary
Ambien	zolpidem	imidazopyridine	Tablet	Treatment of insomnia	Answers will vary
Augmentin	Amoxicillin + clavulanate	penicillin/beta-lactamase inhibitor combination	Tablet and suspension	Bacterial infections	Answers will vary
Avonex	Interferon beta 1a	Amino acid glycoprotein	Lyophilized powder vial and prefilled syringe	Relapsing forms of multiple sclerosis	Answers will vary
Biaxin	clarithromycin	Macrolide	Film tablet and granules for oral suspension	Mild to moderate infections	Answers will vary
Combivir	lamivudine/ zidovudine	Nucleotide reverse transcriptase inhibitor	Tablet	HIV	Answers will vary
Cordarone	amiodarone	Class III antiarrhythmic	Tablet	Arrhythmias	Answers will vary
Detrol LA	tolterodine	Muscarininc receptor antagonist	Extended release capsule	Urinary incontinence	Answers will vary
Dilantin	phenytoin	Related to barbiturates	Extended oral capsule	Epilepsy	Answers will vary
Duragesic	fentanyl	Opioid	Transdermal patch	Management of persistent moderate to severe chronic pain	Answers will vary
Efudex	fluoruracil	Antimetabolite	Cream	Multiple actinic or solar keratoses	Answers will vary
Focalin	dexmethyl- phenidate	CNS stimulant	Tablet	ADHD	Answers will vary
Imuran	azathioprine	Immunosuppressive antimetabolite	Tablets and IV injection	Prevention in renal homotransplanatation and rheumatoid arthritis	Answers will vary
Lexapro	escitalopram	SSRI	Tablet	Depression	Answers will vary
Lovenox	enoxaparin	Heparin	Subcutaneous and Intravenous injection	DVT	Answers will vary
Lupron	leuprolide	Synthetic nonapeptide analog of naturally occurring gonadotropin releasing hormone	Injection	Palliative treatment of advanced prostatic cancer	Answers will vary
Maxalt-MLT	rizatriptan	Selective 5-HT receptor agonist	Oral disintegrating tablets	Migraine headaches	Answers will vary
Oxycontin	oxycodone	Opioid agonist	Controlled release tablets	Moderate to severe pain when continuous around-the-clock therapy is needed	Answers will vary
Procrit	epoetin alpha	Glycoprotein	Injection	Anemia due to chronic renal failure	Answers will vary
Protonix	pantoprazole	Proton pump inhibitor	Delayed release tablets and oral suspension	GERD	Answers will vary

(Continued)

Table 16-1   (Continued)

Brand Name	Generic Name	Drug Classification	Dosage Forms	List Two Indications Of the Medications	List Three Adverse Effects Of the Medication
Stratterra	atomoxetine	Selective norepinephrine reuptake inhibitor	Capsule	ADHD	Answers will vary
Tegretol	carbamazepine	Anticonvulsant	Chewable tablets and suspension	Anticonvulsant	Answers will vary
Wellbutrin	bupropion	Aminoketone antidepressant	Tablet	Antidepressant	Answers will vary
Xopenex	levalbuterol	Beta 2-adrenergic receptor agonist	Inhalation solution	Asthma	Answers will vary

Table 16-2

Brand Name	Retail Pharmacy	Hospital Pharmacy	Long-Term Care Pharmacy	Mail-Order Pharmacy	Federal Pharmacy
Advair	X	X	X	X	X
Ambien	X	X	X	X	X
Augmentin	X	X	X		X
Avonex	X	X	X	X	X
Biaxin	X	X	X		X
Combivir	X	X	X	X	X
Cordarone	X	X	X	X	X
Detrol LA	X	X	X	X	X
Dilantin	X	X	X	X	X
Duragesic	X	X	X		X
Efudex	X	X	X	X	X
Focalin	X	X	X	X	X
Imuran	X	X	X	X	X
Lexapro	X	X	X	X	X
Lovenox	X	X		X	X
Lupron	X			X	X
Maxalt-MLT	X	X	X	X	X
Oxycontin	X	X	X		X
Procrit	X	X	X	X	X
Protonix	X	X	X	X	X
Strattera	X			X	X
Tegretol	X	X	X	X	X
Wellbutrin	X	X	X	X	X
Xopenex	X	X	X	X	X

Chapter 17 Lab

Multiple Choice Answers

1. d—All of the above
   Medications purchased for a pharmacy may be obtained directly through the drug manufacturer, from a company's own warehouse, or through a drug wholesaler.

2. b—DEA Form 222
   A DEA Form 222 is used to transfer Schedule II medications to another pharmacy. There is no official DEA form used to transfer Schedules III, IV, and V substances.

3. b—Biennial
   Federal law requires that a biennial inventory be conducted every 2 years for all pharmacies dispensing controlled substances.
4. a—Inventory management maximizes the costs associated with placing an order
   Proper inventory management should minimize, NOT maximize, the costs associated with placing an order for medications.
5. d—All of the above
   You should always check that the drug received is the same drug with the correct strength as indicated on the invoice (packing slip). The quantity received should be the same as the quantity billed.
6. d—All of the above
   Prime vendors are used because they provide the pharmacy a very high delivery rate of medications on a timely basis; they may provide emergency service for ordering drugs; they often provide the shareware and software to order medications, which includes an electronic ordering device and bar-coded labels; they may offer competitive pricing; and they provide documentation on purchases, pricing information, notification of drug recalls, and various reports.
7. a—Immediately
   A wholesaler should be notified immediately of any merchandise received that is damaged or is not correct with what was ordered or received.
8. d—No DEA form is required
   There is not a DEA form used to order Schedules III, IV, and V medications. These medications are ordered in the same manner as non-controlled substances or OTC medications.
9. d—All of the above
   An individual, pharmaceutical company, governmental agency, or academic institution may bring a new drug to market.
10. d—Submit data demonstrating that the proposed medication is safe to use in clinical studies
    The goal of the sponsor is to bring a new drug entity to market. During this process, it is the responsibility of the sponsor to determine the parameters of the study; initiate and conduct the investigation; and submit data that the proposed drug entity is pure, safe, and effective in the treatment of a specific condition.
11. c—Prophylactic IND
    There are three different types of investigational new drug applications: emergency use IND, investigator IND, and treatment IND. There is no such thing as a prophylactic IND.
12. a—Phase 1
    Phase 1 of the IND utilizes healthy volunteers to determine metabolic and pharmacological actions of the drug, potential side effects due to varying doses, and possible effectiveness of the medication.
13. d—P&T Committee
    The Pharmacy and Therapeutic (P&T) Committee of an institution will determine policies, procedures, and protocol regarding the use of investigational new drugs.
14. c—Class III
    A Class III drug recall is issued in a situation where use of or exposure to a product is not likely to cause adverse health consequences.
15. a—Cold
    The USP has defined "cold" as any temperature not exceeding 8°C (46°F). A "cold" temperature is maintained between 2 and 8°C (36 and 46°F).
16. c—Smaller physical inventories
    A short turnaround time for placing and receiving a drug order allows a pharmacy to maintain smaller physical inventories which can result in higher stock turns (inventory turnover rate).
17. a—Bid
    "Bid" refers to a pharmacy's ability to purchase contract items.
18. d—All of the above
    When stocking shelves, a pharmacy technician should check the expiration date of the medications to prevent short-dated and outdated medications from being dispensed. Rotating the medication so the medication with the shortest time is placed in the front will reduce the possibility of the medication expiring on the shelf. It is important to reread the label to make sure the correct drug and strength are place in the correct place on the shelf. Failure to do so may result in possible shortages of some medications and overages in other medications.
19. d—All of the above
    Just-in-time ordering allows a pharmacy to purchase medications shortly before they are needed. This results in a shorter turnaround time, smaller physical inventories, higher stock turns, and fewer dollars invested in the pharmacy.
20. b—Poor purchasing practices
    Poor purchasing habits result in non-bid purchases of medications.

True/False Answers

1. False. Medication should be placed on the proper location on the shelf, in the safe, or in the refrigerator assigned to the medication. The incoming medication should be placed behind the last item on the shelf.

2. True.

3. True.

4. False. Shortages should be reported immediately to the source of the order. If the pharmacy fails to do so, it may be charged for the medication. If the medication is a controlled substance, the inventory of the medication will not be correct and the pharmacy may face regulatory/legal consequences for failing to maintain proper records.

5. True.

6. False. A DEA Form 224 is used by a pharmacy to apply for a DEA permit to stock and dispense controlled substances.

7. False. A therapeutic equivalent drug is one that contains the same active ingredient(s), strength or concentration, dosage form, and route of administration. A therapeutic interchange is a substitution of one medication that is not generically equivalent but has the same therapeutic effect.

8. False. A "blanket destruction" for controlled substances is for hospitals only.

9. True.

10. True.

11. True.

12. True.

13. True.

14. False. A multiple-dose container for articles intended for parenteral administration only.

15. True.

16. True.

17. False. A group purchasing organization negotiates the prices for an institution. It is the responsibility of the institution to make the actual purchases.

18. True.

19. False. A long-term care facility does not have a DEA number and therefore cannot transfer controlled substances.

20. True.

Apply Your Knowledge Answers

1. Proper inventory management maximizes both profitability and customer service.

2. The pharmacy may not receive exactly what it was billed and therefore the value of the pharmacy will not be correct. Unexpected shortages may occur in the pharmacy of specific medication and therefore affect customer service. Biennial inventories may be incorrect that may cause regulatory problems for the pharmacy.

3. Over ordering and under ordering may occur. Over ordering may cause an excess of medication to be on the shelf. Under ordering may affect customer service and ultimately the profitability of the pharmacy.

4. Medications may expire on the shelf, resulting in lower profits for the pharmacy.

5. A patient may receive an outdated medication and therefore may not experience the proper therapeutic effect of the medication. In some situations, an outdated medication may be fatal to the patient, such as tetracycline. If a board of pharmacy investigator conducts an inspection and finds outdated medication mixed with the regular inventory, the pharmacy will be cited and possibly receive a fine depending on the severity of the infraction.

6. The pharmacy should purchase the ESI Lederle brand of morphine sulfate. $224.80 is saved by ordering this brand.

Drug Manufacturer	Brand Name	Package Size	Quantity	Unit Cost	Extended Cost	Savings
Baxter	Morphine Sulfate	10.00 mL	40	$6.89	$275.60	na
ESI Lederle	Duramorph	10.00 mL	40	$1.27	$ 50.80	$224.80

7. 14.61 inventory turns.

8. First, check the shelf to see if you have any of the indicated medication in stock. If no, the process ends. If yes, pull the recalled medicine off the shelf and place it where it cannot be dispensed. Notify patients who may have received the medication and ask if they experienced any problems. If they did, make notations. If the patients still have any of the medication left, ask them to return it to the pharmacy and provide them with non-recalled medication. Notify the patients' physicians of the situation. Await further directions from the drug manufacturer.

9. Just-in-time ordering minimizes the inventory maintained in the pharmacy.

10. The inventory in the pharmacy should be as low as possible without interrupting a patient's course of treatment or interfere with customer service.

Practice Your Knowledge

Date	Prescription Number	Quantity Dispensed	Invoice Number	Quantity Received	Ending Inventory
June 19			10061908	500	500
June 19	125678	50			450
June 19	125698	25			425
June 20	125789	100			325
June 21	125900	30			295
June 23	126335	60			235
June 23	126338	20			215
June 23	126380	100			115
June 25			123457	500	615
June 26	124899	100			515
June 27	125000	10			505
June 27	125009	20			495

Calculation Corner Answers

Solution

The far right column of the following table indicates the maximum number of bottles or containers you would order but not exceed the maximum quantity.

Drug	Package Size	Qty. On Hand	Max. Qty.	Qty. Ordered
Amoxil 500 mg	500 caps/btl	750 caps	1500 caps	1 btl
Lotrisone Cream	15 g/tube	3 tubes	1 tube	2 tubes
Cephalexin 500 mg	100 caps/btl	125 caps	600 caps	3 btls
Ortho Novum 1/35	6 × 28 tabs/box	224 tabs	672 tabs	2 boxes
Albuterol Inhaler	17 g/inhaler	5 inhalers	17 inhalers	12 inhalers
Robitussin AC	4 fl oz/btl	12 btls	10 btls	0 btls
Calan SR 240 mg	100 tabs/btl	450 tabs	625 tabs	1 btl
Timoptic 0.025%	15 mL/btl	2 btls	4 btls	2 btls
Fluoxetine 20 mg	30 caps/btl	12.5 btls	19 btls	6 btls
Naproxyn 500 mg	100 tabs/btl	3.75 btls	5.25 btls	1 btl

Pharmacy Facts—Research Answers

Table 17-1

Brand Name	Generic Name	Strength	Schedule	List One Indication of the Medication	List Three Adverse Effects of the Medication
Ambien	zolpidem	5 and 10 mg tablets	IV	Short term treatment of insomnia	Answers will vary
Ativan	lorazepam	0.5 mg, 1mg and 2 mg tablets	IV	Anxiety disorders	Answers will vary
Concerta	methylphenidate	18 mg, 27 mg, 36 mg and 54 mg	II	ADHD	Answers will vary

(Continued)

Table 17-1   (Continued)

Brand Name	Generic Name	Strength	Schedule	List One Indication of the Medication	List Three Adverse Effects of the Medication
Dalmane	flurazepam	15 mg and 30 mg	IV	Insomnia	Answers will vary
Darvocet N-100	Propoxyphene and acetaminophen	100 mg/325 mg	IV	Mild to moderate pain	Answers will vary
Demerol	meperidine	50 and 100 mg	II	Moderate to severe pain	Answers will vary
Dilaudid	hydromorphone	8 mg	II	Pain management in patients where an opioid analgesic is appropriate	Answers will vary
Hycodan	hydrocodone/homatropine	5 mg	III	Symptomatic relief of cough	Answers will vary
Lunesta	escopiclone	1 mg, 2 mg and 3 mg	IV	Treatment of insomnia	Answers will vary
Percocet 5	oxycodone/acetaminophen	5mg/325 mg	II	Moderate to moderately severe pain	Answers will vary
Phenobarbital	phenobarbital	30 mg, 60 mg and 100 mg	IV	Sedative, hypnotic, preanesthetic and treatment of tonic-clonic local seizures	Answers will vary
Ritalin	methylphenidate	5 mg, 10 mg and 20 mg	II	ADHD	Answers will vary
Robitussin AC	Guaifenesin/codeine	100 mg/10 mg	IV	Cough due to minor throat and bronchial irritation	Answers will vary
Serax	oxazepam	10 mg, 15 mg and 30 mg	IV	Anxiety disorders	Answers will vary
Stadol NS	butorphanol	10 mg/mL	IV	Management of pain when the use of an opioid analgesic is appropriate	Answers will vary
Tylenol with Codeine #3	acetaminophen/codeine	300 mg/30 mg	III	Relief of mild to moderate pain	Answers will vary
Valium	diazepam	2 mg, 5 mg and 10 mg	IV	Anxiety	Answers will vary
Vicodin	hydrocodone/acetaminophen	5 mg/500 mg	III	Moderate to moderately severe pain	Answers will vary
Vicodin ES	hydrocodone/acetaminophen	7.5 mg/750 mg	III	Moderate to moderately severe pain	Answers will vary
Xanax	alprazolam	0.25 mg, 0.5 mg, 1 mg and 2 mg	IV	Anxiety disorders	Answers will vary

Chapter 18 Lab

Multiple Choice Answers

1. a—Didactic courses
   Students primarily attend lectures and take exams in the didactic course of the pharmacy technician program.
2. b—Laboratory
   A mock pharmacy environment is often employed in the laboratory courses in the pharmacy technician program.
3. d—American Society of Heath-System Pharmacists
   ASHP is responsible for accreditation for pharmacy technician programs.
4. d—All of the above
   Networking involves meeting colleagues, participating in professional events, and meeting potential employers.
5. b—Arriving on time
   Arriving on time constitutes professional behavior.
6. d—All of the above are components of the resume
   Contact information, employment history, and education are all components of the resume.

7. d—Salary history
   Salary history is not included in a cover letter.
8. c—Immunization records
   Immunization records are not part of the personal portfolio.
9. d—All of the above
   To prepare for an interview a pharmacy technician should research the prospective employer's organization, determine responses to appropriate interview questions, and draft a few questions to ask the interviewer.
10. d—Chewing gum
    Chewing gum should not be brought to the interview.
11. d—Attempting to entertain the interviewers is not appropriate during the interview.
12. c—Arrange to arrive at least 10 minutes early
    Arranging to arrive at least 10 minutes early is a good strategy to employ for a job interview.
13. c—It can affect your relationship with a future employer
    Attitude can affect your relationship with a future employer.
14. c—Call the interviewer(s) daily until you are offered the job
    Following the interview you should not call the interviewer(s) daily until you are offered the job.
15. d—Sunglasses
    Sunglasses should not be worn during an interview.
16. d—All of the above
    When answering questions during an interview, it is important to maintain eye contact, speak clearly and be concise, and display a professional attitude.
17. c—When would you be able to start work?
    When you would be able to start work is a appropriate question for an interviewer to ask an applicant.
18. d—All of the above
    You should be able to answer all of these questions.
19. b—Embellish your responses
    You should not embellish your responses when completing an application for employment.
20. d—All of the above
    In preparation for applying for a job, the pharmacy technician should be prepared to take a drug screening test, complete an employment application, and provide proof of education/certification/registration.
21. d—a and b
    In preparation for applying for a job, the pharmacy technician should also be prepared to take a pre-employment physical exam and provide proof of immunizations.
22. a—Learn from the experience to determine how to improve your chances in the future.
    In the event you are not offered the position you applied for, you should learn from the experience to determine how to improve your chances in the future.

23. c—Cover letter
    When mailing your resume it should be accompanied by a cover letter.
24. a—Fax cover sheet
    When faxing your resume to a prospective employer, you should include a fax cover sheet.
25. b—Not applicable
    N/A on a job application means not applicable.

Apply Your Knowledge Answers

1. A—It is appropriate to send a cover letter with a resume for an advertised position.
2. U—An emailed resume should always be accompanied by a cover letter or email message
3. A—It is appropriate to be asked by a prospective employer if you are certified
4. A—It is appropriate to be asked by a prospective employer to take a pre-employment physical examination.
5. U—It is inappropriate for a prospective employer to ask about your ethnic background.
6. A—It is appropriate and advisable to research the prospective employer's company on the internet to prepare for an interview.
7. U—It is inappropriate to submit an application for employment with some items left blank.
8. U—It is inappropriate and unprofessional to insult the interviewer after being told that you did not get the position for which you applied.
9. A—It is appropriate and advisable to practice answering potential interview questions in a mock setting with your classmates.
10. A—It is appropriate to ask your pharmacy technician instructor for advice prior to going for a job interview.
11. U—It is never appropriate to embellish or make false statements on a resume.
12. A—It is appropriate to refuse to provide information to a prospective employer regarding your religious affiliation.
13. U—It is inappropriate to refuse to submit to a pre-employment drug test.
14. U—It is inappropriate to interrupt the prospective employer during the interview.
15. U—It is inappropriate to answer your cell phone during an interview.

Calculation Corner Answers

Solution

Calculate your salary adjusted to include fringe benefits:

$32, 000 \times 0.29 = \$9,280$
$32,000 + 9,280 = \$41,280$

Your salary including fringe benefits would be $41,280.

Chapter 19 Lab

Multiple Choice Answers

1. c—PTCB
   The Pharmacy Technician Certification Board is an organization responsible for certification of pharmacy technicians.
2. b—State board of pharmacy
   The state board of pharmacy is responsible for registration or licensure of pharmacy technicians.
3. c—ASHP
   The American Society of Health-System Pharmacists is responsible for accreditation of pharmacy technician programs.
4. c—PTEC
   The Pharmacy Technician Educators Council was established for pharmacy technician educators.
5. b—Must complete a pharmacy technician program
   Completion of a pharmacy technician program is not a requirement for the Pharmacy Technician Certification Examination.
6. b—Certified pharmacy technician
   CPhT means certified pharmacy technician.
7. d—The exam must be taken again
   It is not required to take the exam again for renewal of the CPhT.
8. d—AAPT
   The American Association of Pharmacy Technicians is not a certifying agency for pharmacy technicians.
9. b—NPTA
   The National Pharmacy Technician Association was founded specifically for pharmacy technicians.
10. b—ACPE
    The Accreditation Council for Pharmacy Education accredits/approves continuing education providers.
11. c—Skip your breaks and lunch periods
    Skipping your breaks and lunch periods is not an appropriate stress management technique.
12. b—Try to do everything at once
    Trying to do everything at once is not an appropriate time management technique.
13. b—Performance appraisal form
    Another term for employee evaluation form is performance appraisal form.
14. d—Intelligence
    Intelligence is not criteria for evaluation and is not likely to appear on a pharmacy technician's performance appraisal form.
15. b—0.1 CEU
    One hour of continuing education credit is identified as 0.1 CEU.
16. a—ACPE
    The Accreditation Council for Pharmacy Education accredits continuing education providers.
17. d—All of the above
18. c—The employee's personality is the primary criterion for evaluation
    The employee's performance is the primary criterion for evaluation.
19. a—0.1
    At least 0.1 CEU of pharmacy law is needed to maintain the PTCB certification.
20. d—All of the above

Matching Answers

1. D   2. A   3. B   4. E   5. C

True/False Answers

1. True.
2. True.
3. False. The focus of the NPTA is primarily the practice of pharmacy technicians.
4. True.
5. False. The PTCB is an organization that certifies pharmacy technicians.
6. True.
7. True.
8. False. The pharmacy technician's certificate or registration card must be displayed in the pharmacy where the technician works.
9. True.
10. True.

Calculation Corner Answers

Solution

1. Knowing that 0.1 continuing education units (CEUs) is equivalent to 1 hour of credit, how many hours of credit have you earned?

   0.1 CEU = 1 credit hour
   Total CEU = 0.2 + 0.3 + 0.1 + 0.2
   = 0.8 CEU or
   = 8 credit hours

   You have earned 8 credit hours.

2. How many more hours do you need to earn to meet the continuing education requirements to renew certification?

   Total hours required = 20 hours
   Earned hours = 8 hours
   Hours needed = 20 − 8
   = 12 hours

   You need to earn 12 more hours to meet the certification renewal requirements.

Credits

PTCB Knowledge Statements, used with permission, Pharmacy Technician Certification Board.

Chapter opener

1: © Total Care Programming, Inc.;
2: © The McGraw-Hill Companies, Inc./Christopher Kerrigan, photographer;
3: © Comstock Images/Jupiter Images/RF;
4: Hinter/Nagle, Pharmacology: An Introduction, 5e, © The McGraw-Hill Companies;
5: © Stockdisc/PunchStock/RF;
6: Hinter/Nagle, Pharmacology: An Introduction, 5e, © The McGraw-Hill Companies;
7: © Royalty-Free/CORBIS;
8: © The McGraw-Hill Companies, Inc./Jill Braaten, photographer;
9: © Royalty-Free/CORBIS;
10: © Stockdisc/Punchstock/RF;
11: Courtesy Total Care Programming;
12: © Royalty-Free/CORBIS;
13: Courtesy Total Care Programming;
14: Courtesy Total Care Programming;
15: © Ryan McVay/Getty Images/RF;
16: © The McGraw-Hill Companies, Inc./Rick Brady, photographer;
17: Courtesy Total Care Programming;
18: © C. Sherburne/Photo Link/Getty Images/RF;
19: © Stockbyte/Punchstock/RF.